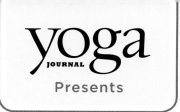

RESTORATIVE YOGA FOR LIFE

A Relaxing Way to De-stress,
Re-energize, and Find Balance

Gail Boorstein Grossman, E-RYT 500, CYKT

Adams Media
New York   London   Toronto   Sydney   New Delhi

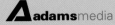

Adams Media
An Imprint of Simon & Schuster, Inc.
57 Littlefield Street
Avon, Massachusetts 02322

For information about special discounts for bulk purchases, please contact Simon & Schuster Special Sales at 1-866-506-1949 or business@simonandschuster.com.

The Simon & Schuster Speakers Bureau can bring authors to your live event. For more information or to book an event contact the Simon & Schuster Speakers Bureau at 1-866-248-3049 or visit our website at www.simonspeakers.com.

Chakra icon drawings provided by Dvora Troshane. Chakra illustration on page 24 © Peter Hermes Furian/123RF. All other photography by Deana Travers, Home Town Photo.

Manufactured in the United States of America

10 9 8 7 6 5

Library of Congress Cataloging-in-Publication Data has been applied for.

ISBN 978-1-4405-7520-4
ISBN 978-1-4405-7521-1(ebook)

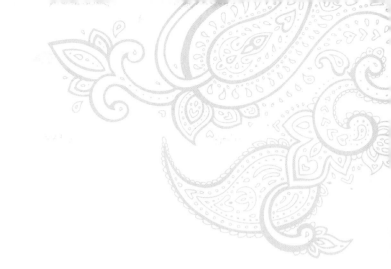

DEDICATION

*To my mother and my aunt, who inspire me every day
to be like the wonderful women they were.*

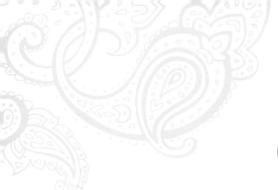

CONTENTS

PART 3

THE SEQUENCES. 124

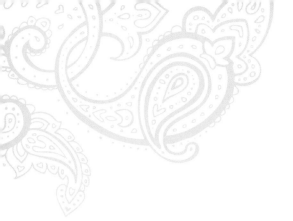

PREFACE

When I first began practicing yoga, I was working in a completely different job, was commuting to the city, and had two young children at home. I came to yoga at the urging of my acupuncturist who suggested that it might help heal a swollen lymph node. I had originally gone to my regular doctor and was told that it was nothing to worry about, but that answer didn't sit well with me. I knew there was a better way to connect with myself and make myself feel better and I thought yoga might be it. I started taking class once a week, as that was all I could fit into my schedule, but soon started feeling that if I didn't practice I didn't feel as good in my body. Before I knew it, I was studying to become a yoga teacher.

The knowledge shared in this book has been passed on to me from my teachers, in the same way that yoga has been shared for many years. There are many teachers of restorative yoga, but perhaps the most well-known figure in the field is Judith Hanson Lasater, my teacher. She wrote the book *Relax and Renew* in 1995, and it is a wonderful resource to yoga students and teachers alike. Judith, who trains hundreds of yoga teachers a year in her Relax and Renew programs, has been an inspiring teacher, as she truly lives her yoga. She has healed herself many times with this practice, and many others as well. Not only is she a yoga teacher, she is also a physical therapist, and I feel very fortunate to have learned from someone who has such a wealth of knowledge. Because Judith has shared this practice with others, because she believes it to be her dharma (life's work), many people will benefit from this incredibly healing practice.

I have also been fortunate to learn from Cora Wen, a gifted teacher who is a longtime assistant to Judith. Cora's love of restorative yoga has only deepened my appreciation for all the multitudes of therapeutic applications it has to offer. I hope to pass these postures on to you and provide an understanding of how you can benefit from the deeply rewarding practice of restorative yoga. I'm happy that you've chosen to learn more about this practice!

So why am I writing this book? Why have I chosen to pass my knowledge of restorative yoga along to you? It really wasn't a choice. Life is like that sometimes; things just keep showing up until you pay attention to them. It's how I became a yoga teacher, opened a yoga studio, and studied with whom I studied. This book came to be because this book's time has come. Restorative yoga is becoming better known because there are more and more people like me out there sharing these teachings, so that people can feel good! Feeling good is our human right. This book includes associated information beyond restorative yoga; when you start the practice, you may not want to know more, but when you're ready, it will be there, waiting for you. I hope you enjoy the journey.

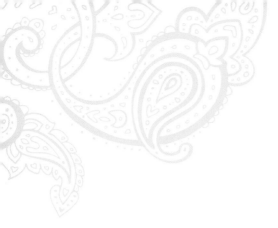

INTRODUCTION

"There is only one corner of the universe you can be certain of improving, and that's your own self."

—Aldous Huxley, British novelist

You may have done some yoga in the past or practice it regularly, or perhaps you've never done yoga before. If you have done very little or no yoga, this book will help clarify what yoga is in general, and what restorative yoga is in particular. If you are familiar with yoga, this book will offer you a better understanding of what restorative yoga is, and how it is both similar and different from "regular" yoga. You will also learn more about how restorative yoga's deeply healing benefits can enhance your yoga repertoire. But whether you're a beginner or an experienced yoga practitioner, you will find that the practice of restorative yoga can help you to live a long and comfortable life in the body you have. Its beauty is that everyone can do it, and everyone *should.* Since you only have one body, you might as well treat it in the best way you can!

So just what *is* restorative yoga and . . .

• Is it yoga?

• Is it therapy?

• Is it restful?

The answer is yes, yes, yes, and much more!

Most people know that the pace of modern life has led to many problems with our health, and at the root of most of these problems is stress. Restorative yoga focuses on undoing that stress. It functions like the more active styles of yoga, but typically works on a deeper level. Since restorative yoga poses are held longer than more active yoga poses, they have the time to penetrate your body's systems—including your mind—to create significant shifts in both physical and mental health. It is becoming a more popular practice, and for good reason!

Throughout *Yoga Journal Presents Restorative Yoga for Life* you'll find the general information, poses, and sequences needed to practice restorative yoga. The information here is comprehensive, though there is a suggested reading list in the back if you want to learn further. In Part 1, you will learn about the history of the practice, its benefits, and the props you need to get yourself set up and ready to practice at home (or anywhere!). Part 2 gives you step-by-step information on the actual poses that make up the practice. Each pose entry contains detailed information on how to set up the pose, which is very important because restorative yoga poses are typically more involved and take longer to set up than "regular" yoga poses. You'll also find instructions on how to do the breathing exercises and visualizations that are the bedrock of any yoga practice. Yoga is fueled by breath first and foremost, and restorative yoga is no different. Keep these exercises and visualizations in the back of your mind as you do any of the poses in Part 2. In Part 3 you'll learn a variety of restorative yoga pose sequences that can target common health issues. The gentle manner of restorative yoga has proven time and again to be very effective in helping people restore themselves to health. You'll also learn how to create sequences of your own.

So whether you are only starting out in yoga, a seasoned practitioner, or even just curious about restorative yoga, this book is a great place to get started. Let's begin!

PART 1

WHAT IS RESTORATIVE YOGA?

"Healing is a matter of time, but it is sometimes also a matter of opportunity."

—Hippocrates, ancient Greek physician

There are many styles of yoga, each founded in certain aims and goals of practitioners both ancient and modern. But what is restorative yoga? In this section, you'll be introduced to the history of this very recent yoga practice and explore its roots. You'll also learn about restorative yoga's many benefits—physical and psychological—that have contributed to the popularity of the practice, and how you can use restorative yoga to feel better in your body, calmer in your mind, and happier in your life. But just learning about restorative yoga isn't enough. You also need to educate yourself about the philosophies, related practices, and bodies of knowledge that support yoga in general. Knowing a little about Ayurveda and the chakra system, in particular, can help you gain a deeper understanding of your body. So be sure to read all of the information in this first part carefully before you begin—there is a lot to know about restorative yoga!

CHAPTER 1

HISTORY OF RESTORATIVE YOGA

"Be at least as interested in what goes on inside you as what happens outside. If you get the inside right, the outside will fall into place."

—Eckhart Tolle, writer and public speaker

You may know that there are many different styles of yoga. If you are someone who likes to sweat when you exercise, you may want to practice a more vigorous style of yoga, such as Ashtanga or Power Vinyasa. There is also Bikram yoga, which, by virtue of being practiced in a very heated room, will make you sweat. If you prefer a gentler style of yoga, you may want to practice gentle yoga, Hatha yoga, Kripalu yoga, or Iyengar yoga; while you may still sweat in these classes, they are less vigorous.

In this chapter you'll learn about the relatively new practice of restorative yoga, which is unique in that it uses props to hold you in poses for a period of time, as opposed to moving at a faster pace. You see, yoga is so much more than physical exercise. It incorporates both a philosophy of how to live and physical postures that you can practice. Yoga not only increases flexibility and strength, but will also help you quiet your mind and engender a deeper connection to yourself. But what really makes restorative yoga special? Read on.

WHAT IS RESTORATIVE YOGA?

Restorative yoga is a deeply relaxing style of yoga practice. It is a _receptive_ practice, not an _active_ practice. Unlike the more active styles of yoga where poses "flow" into one another, in restorative yoga poses are held from five to as long as twenty minutes. During this time, you are held in "shapes" while being supported with blankets, blocks, or bolsters (pillows). The shapes emulate the forms of some more active poses found in Ashtanga, Vinyasa, or Iyengar such as a back bend, forward bend, twist, or inversion. When you are in the poses you are completely supported in a particular shape, which helps achieve the desired benefit—it could open up your lungs, release tension in your lower back, or any of the other benefits discussed later in Chapter 2—as well as help you feel comfortable enough to "let go."

In any style of yoga, part of the practice is about letting go of the ego. Restorative yoga is no different. Yoga teaches patience, devotion, and faith. When you apply the teachings both on and beyond the mat, your mind is better able to adjust to the stresses of everyday life and is brought into harmony with your body. In restorative yoga, the body and mind are brought into balance, and begin to "talk" to each other. When you practice this type of yoga, you enter into a state of deep relaxation. It is here that you can "let go" of those deep holding patterns in your body and find a state of balance that will allow your body to heal. Look at it as if you were a flower. You start with good soil (the foundation), add sunshine and water, and the flower opens into a beautiful bloom. You are like a flower; you need the right environment to allow yourself to unfold and become the best version of yourself. Restorative yoga is that environment.

We often forget that sometimes we need to just take time to relax. We are not human "doings," we are human beings. If you think that there is no way you can relax, you need restorative yoga more than you know. As with meditation practice, it takes time to train the mind to find some quiet. In fact, some people find the practice of restorative yoga to be the most difficult of all yoga practices because it is so hard to be still. Your body may be at rest, but that doesn't mean your mind will follow! Be prepared for when the mind starts to ramble. This is the moment where you will need to call upon yourself to find stillness, what practicing yoga is all about. You can equate the process to training a puppy. You tell it to sit and stay; it gets up two seconds later. You take the puppy back to where it started and try again. This time it may stay a little longer, until eventually it stays until you tell it to move. In restorative yoga, we build up to being able to stay longer. This is the kind of stamina that every one of us could use.

Restorative yoga is best done daily for maximum benefit, but can be done as little as once a week to see results. Restorative postures can also be integrated into a regular yoga practice to give greater balance to a more active practice and lifestyle. I assure you, once you get the hang of restorative yoga, you will fall in love!

YOGIC WISDOM

Yoga is often passed on from teacher to student, so use caution when you begin. If you will not have supervision it is always wise to consult your physician first. This book does not replace a medical professional!

HOW DID RESTORATIVE YOGA BEGIN?

Now that you know what restorative yoga is, it's important for you to know how the practice began. The development of restorative yoga poses began in 1937 with B.K.S. Iyengar, a master yoga teacher from Pune, India.

Iyengar learned yoga from his yoga teacher and brother-in-law, Tirumalai Krishnamacharya. Iyengar was a sickly teenager, and yoga helped him to regain his strength. He soon become a star pupil and actually replaced another one of Krishnamacharya's students in a yoga competition. Back then, it was commonplace to have yoga competitions to show the public the skill of these students and educate the public on the practice. Restorative yoga grew out of Iyengar's need to find therapeutic poses that would help him heal and restore his physical body.

Iyengar began teaching yoga at the age of eighteen. While teaching, Iyengar noticed his students straining in postures that could result in injury and pain. When people first come to yoga, they tend to bring the "no pain no gain" mentality along with their mats. In traditional yoga, practitioners challenge themselves to advance, and often try to advance at a fast pace, which can often cause injury. This is precisely what Iyengar was noticing in his classes—people pushing themselves too far, and causing injury. While pain is inevitable in any practice where you are working with your body, you never want to cause injury. Unlike the more active styles of yoga, restorative yoga's philosophy looks a lot different. Here, you learn to push yourself more gently—without a competitive attitude. Here, it's "no pain = gain."

This idea is what led Iyengar to incorporate props into his yoga practice so that poses could be modified and practiced without strain, helping people recover from injury, overworking, and illness in a therapeutic way. Props are exactly what they sound like: pillows called bolsters, blocks, chairs, the wall, blankets—all of which prop you up in positions that help you hold a healing shape for a period of time. Restorative yoga poses originated in the Iyengar tradition, using props to help each individual student find the alignment of each specific posture that works best for his or her body in any given moment. As time went on, Iyengar traveled to the West to share his teachings with others. When people began to understand the benefits of yoga, they traveled from all over the world to study with him. Until his death in 2014 at the age of 95, Iyengar certified teachers in his style of yoga, and those teachers disseminated the teachings in their own countries.

To this day people travel to India to learn from the Iyengar family, to recover from injury and from both physical and emotional illnesses. Iyengar's son Prashant and daughter Geeta both have carried on his teachings, as has his granddaughter Abhijata.

Yoga has a long, rich history, a history that we in the West are only beginning to understand. The information presented here will help introduce you to the practice, and hopefully inspire you to learn more about its history and philosophies. Restorative yoga is a relatively new style of yoga, and is becoming popular because it addresses the ills of our fast-paced society so effectively. It gives the body a real sense of the healing power of *just being still*, which is actually the heart of the practice of yoga and meditation. Practice, however, is the real first step. It is for that reason you are here, so read on! But first, let's cover the benefits of restorative yoga.

CHAPTER 2

BENEFITS OF RESTORATIVE YOGA

"And in the end, it's not the years in your life that count. It's the life in your years."

—Abraham Lincoln, U.S. President

The best way to describe the benefits of restorative yoga is to perhaps ask what *aren't* the benefits of restorative yoga? If you have suffered from stress, trauma, injury, or illness, this practice can help you heal. If you are just a regular person, with a normal amount of stress in your life, and want to continue to feel good in your body, this practice will help you maintain that well-being. Ultimately, everyone wants to feel at ease in his or her own body, and to achieve a sense of union with their true nature. This is the main "goal" of yoga, and it is what we all deserve to achieve in our lifetime.

You see, both physical and mental activities influence each other, creating imbalances in the body. Restorative yoga is a process that leads to self-discovery. It helps bring the mind and body into balance by creating the mind's awareness of the body's limitations; as you become more connected to your physical body, you are able to better connect to your emotional body, and discover what ails you.

In Part 3, you'll find pose sequences that will help you deal with specific injuries, illnesses, and various emotional challenges. But before you start practicing these sequences, you need to know more about the benefits of yoga in general, and how restorative yoga can help you achieve balance. Read on to learn more!

YOGA, IN GENERAL

Before we can begin talking about the specific benefits of restorative yoga, it's important for you to realize the ways in which any sort of yoga can help you manage and balance both your physical body and emotional being. Yoga can be looked at as a tree with eight limbs. These limbs are a culmination of thousands of years of wisdom and knowledge of ancient yogis. Each limb in itself is a set of guidelines.

First, there are the Yamas and the Niyamas (together referred to by some as the "Ten Commandments"), which offer moral and ethical guidelines on how to conduct yourself in your dealings with others, as well as self-discipline. Asana is a third limb, containing the postures of yoga. Pranayama is a fourth limb, which contains the breathing techniques of yoga. These first four limbs help us to refine who we are in this world: how we show up, how we interact with others, and how we manage the bodies we have been given.

YOGIC WISDOM

The eight-limbed path of yoga is called Ashtanga ("ashta" meaning "eight" and "tanga" meaning "limbs"; it is not to be confused with the style of yoga called Ashtanga yoga that was created by Pattabhi Jois) and was first put to paper by a sage named Patanjali, many hundreds of years ago.

It's important to note that yoga is not a linear process: Sometimes we need to explore our inner world to affect our outer world. The next four limbs—Pratyahara, Dharana, Dhyana, and Samadhi—refer to the refinement of our inner world. Pratyahara means "withdrawal from the senses," and teaches us that when we withdraw our attention from outer stimuli, we draw closer to a clearer, more objective picture of ourselves. This leads to better concentration, which is what Dharana teaches. It is hard to concentrate, in this day and age, with so much drawing our attention away (all the electronic gadgets, etc.). When we learn to concentrate, we work toward retraining the brain and bringing it under control. This perfected concentration drops you into a flow of experience called meditation or Dhyana. (These two limbs, Dharana and Dhyana, are often confused, but you need to be skillful at concentration before you can experience true meditation.) The final limb is Samadhi. It is believed that when we practice the philosophical and physical aspects of yoga, we can experience a feeling of bliss. It's important to note that there are many levels of bliss in yogic texts, but for the purpose of simplifying, bliss is the feeling of being in the flow, like when you are so wrapped up in an activity that you lose track of space and time.

Now that you have a better understanding of what yoga is about, you can learn how restorative yoga in particular will benefit you on both a physical and psychological level.

PHYSICAL BENEFITS

It's important to understand that most of the things you do in your daily life can lead to imbalances in the body. The repetition of everyday life, in both physical and nonphysical ways, can send our bodies out of alignment very easily. Whenever you move, you create opportunities for your body to become out of alignment. Active people often create imbalances in their body from overuse—for example, golfers tend to have back and arm issues. Simple motions we do every day can cause imbalances, too—for example, mothers are prone to back issues because they often carry a baby on one hip. However, the same opportunities for imbalance exist even when you don't move. Inactive people foster imbalances through the "use it or lose it" concept: Spending long hours at a desk will cause hunched shoulders and tight neck muscles.

For those with moderate to severe physical impairments, no matter how they're caused, physical activity can become nearly impossible. People suffering from injuries such as a torn rotator cuff, torn tendon, or tennis elbow can find a traditional yoga practice impossible. Sufferers of chronic diseases such as arthritis and neuropathy of the

YOGIC WISDOM

It is debated whether Samadhi, the bliss that is the culmination of yoga, can be reached without perfected practice of all eight limbs of yoga philosophy. From a Tantric perspective, everything in the universe is interrelated and interconnected, and therefore we can. From a Vedantic perspective, the climb to Samadhi is more linear, and we cannot. There are many books that you can read to further research these yogic schools of thought. My favorites include Tantra: The Path of Ecstasy *by Georg Feuerstein,* Tantra: Cult of the Feminine *by Andre van Lysebeth, and* American Veda: From Emerson and the Beatles to Yoga and Meditation—How Indian Spirituality Changed the West *by Philip Goldberg.*

limbs can also find physical activity unbearable. Restorative yoga helps to counteract all of these movements, and "restore" the body to balance. The practice is beneficial because restorative yoga works in a passive, not active, manner, and it places your body in shapes that are effective on both a physical and emotional level, without strain. Even if yoga is not your usual thing, restorative yoga is a great addition to your physical well-being. Many of us do not take the time to restore our muscles; we just work them until one day they tell you where to go! Practicing restorative yoga can keep you from injuring yourself. It is a great way to loosen the muscles that get tight from overuse. In Part 3, you'll learn specific restorative yoga sequences that help heal specific physical (and emotional) ailments, but the following are just some of the overall physical benefits of restorative yoga:

- **Restores you after surgery:** Because restorative yoga is restful, you can regain energy when you practice it, which will help you heal. Certain poses and sequences can also help you recover from specific surgeries.

- **Prevents disease:** Restorative yoga is known to help prevent many diseases such as heart disease and diabetes. It is incredibly beneficial, because the poses lower cortisol levels in the system. When relaxation is induced and cortisol lowers, blood pressure levels likewise lower, as well as glucose levels.

- **Helps relieve women's issues:** Restorative yoga can be therapeutic for pregnancy, menstruation, and menopause. There are many side effects of menopause that have to do with shifting hormonal levels, which restorative yoga can help balance. With menstruation, not only are you dealing with hormones, but also physical discomfort that comes from bloating and cramps. Restorative

yoga can be a wonderfully therapeutic way to treat that discomfort, but vigorous poses and inversions should be avoided during the time that you are bleeding. Restorative yoga is also a very helpful practice when you feel tired or weighed down during pregnancy. This practice is safe and beneficial to your energy, but you shouldn't practice vigorous yoga or breath retention while pregnant, or poses involving deep twists or unsupported inversions.

- **Helps relieve cold and flu symptoms:** If you suffer from a cold, which typically manifests as upper respiratory congestion and coughing, rest is encouraged and restorative yoga is a great practice supporting this. You can heal faster when you are well rested, which is one of the benefits of restorative yoga, and there are also specific poses that help relieve sinus pressure, increase circulation, and help you breathe more easily.

- **Provides headache relief:** Headaches can be caused by tension or a pinched nerve near the spine; they also can stem from migraines, which are typically vascular and can occur for women more than men due to their menses. Headaches can be helped with restorative poses, especially ones that help induce a deep state of relaxation, as we know headaches can be caused by anxiety. There are also poses that passively stretch certain muscles that may constrict blood flow and cause a headache. Applying pressure by wrapping the head with a large ace bandage, or placing a sandbag on the forehead, is also very helpful in headache relief.

- **Provides relief from carpal tunnel syndrome:** This painful syndrome presents itself when the carpal ligament in the wrist becomes compressed, which can cause pain, tingling, numbness, or weakness in the wrist or hand. Carpal tunnel syndrome is often triggered by the overuse of your wrists, from typing at the computer or other straining postures that affect your shoulders and arm alignment. Restorative yoga doesn't put pressure on the wrists and is perfect for people with carpal tunnel. Poses that help treat carpal tunnel look to realign the body so that you learn to carry yourself in a way that eases the tension in the wrists. A simple shift in alignment can make a big difference.

- **Helps reduce obesity:** When high-intensity aerobic activity (proven to burn calories and reduce fat) is just not practical, restorative yoga can be a surprising answer to helping overweight men and women still achieve weight loss. Studies have shown that restorative yoga reduces the level of cortisol in your system. If you have excessive body fat, restorative yoga makes a very nice adjunct to a more active yoga practice. There have been studies showing that you can actually lose more fat from practicing restorative yoga than practicing a more vigorous yoga. When cortisol production in the body is lowered, the amount of glucose being created in the body is likewise decreased. Glucose creates fat, especially belly fat, which can lead to other diseases as well. If you reduce stress, you reduce cortisol and then glucose, which leads to weight loss. Certain poses are more effective than others to achieve a sense of relaxation.

- **Relieves sciatica:** When the sciatic nerve is irritated, it becomes inflamed and creates pain that starts at the buttocks and radiates all the way down the leg. Many restorative poses create traction that takes pressure off the nerve.

- **Relieves symptoms from spinal cord injuries:** If you suffer from a spinal cord injury, the damage of some of the fibers in the spinal cord causes a degree of loss of muscle function. Restorative

yoga and breathing techniques are very helpful in improving muscle function.

- **Gives you more energy:** Resting is underrated by our society. In fact, most people are sleep deprived, and try to make up for it by drinking caffeinated beverages, which in turn keeps them from being able to sleep, and so on. It creates a vicious cycle. When you practice restorative yoga, you relax the nervous system and create a state of rest in the body, without actually sleeping. A simple pose like Legs Up the Wall (both with or without a bolster) for twenty minutes can make you feel much more energized!

In addition to all of these amazing benefits, restorative yoga can also help reduce physical tension and pain.

A Note about Pain

Pain is a great teacher. When I herniated a disc in my lumbar spine, I kept saying to myself, "There is a reason for this." There was. In the process of recovery, I learned so much about herniation and how to treat it through restorative yoga, and have been able to pass that valuable firsthand knowledge on to my students. Pain, being a great teacher in and of itself, has made me a better yoga teacher.

> **YOGIC WISDOM**
>
> *You may have heard of a herniated disc referred to as a slipped disc or a bulging disc. It happens when the disc protrudes beyond its normal space, putting pressure on the spinal cord or nerves. The pain caused by this out-of-place disc may radiate from the back all the way down to the foot, or from the neck all the way down the arm. Vigorous yoga is not recommended in a situation like this, but restorative practice is supportive, and you can do as much or as little as you can handle.*

Many times the place where you feel pain in your body is not actually the spot from which the pain emanates. Understanding this will be important when you develop a plan for your restorative yoga practice. The good news is that the practice of restorative yoga is very effective at supporting overall health and well-being. When you address the "whole," the "parts" follow. Many times restorative yoga can help heal specific causes of pain without you actually having to be specific in your approach.

Injury and illness can trigger "pain" in your body—that is something you cannot control. However, how you handle the pain or respond to the pain you feel is something that you can control. Pain does not have to control you! You have more power than you realize. If you can understand how to decrease your "pain response"—the sensations you feel, the thoughts you have about the pain, the emotions, coping mechanisms you use, etc.—you can manage your pain to the point where you are actually controlling it. Once you begin to handle the challenge of dealing with pain, you can handle the pain in a much better, healthier way. Furthermore, when you work to discover the root cause (or causes) of the recurring pain in your body, learn what worsens that pain, and address the root causes, you can begin to *truly* heal. Restorative yoga can be key in this healing. By teaching you how to truly relax and let go, restorative yoga helps you learn how to release your responses to pain, and create a new relationship to healing.

PSYCHOLOGICAL BENEFITS

Our bodies like to thrive in a state of ease. Ease means less tension and stress. When we have less of that we have more comfort in our bodies and more calm minds. Dis-ease can cause disease, and can lead to many of the physical issues that restorative yoga can help heal and prevent, including heart disease, obesity, headaches, cancer, and more. When you take the time to practice restorative yoga, you can heal from these things, but better yet, you can keep these things from ever becoming an issue. How? Through restorative yoga's psychological benefits.

The psychological benefits of yoga are well documented. For example, it establishes mindfulness that leads to better life choices and consequently a happier state of being; it enhances patience, which leads to better relationships—the list is long. Restorative yoga offers all the same benefits as any other style of yoga, but it also offers psychological benefits that come specifically out of this unique practice. Since the poses (discussed in Chapter 5) are held for long lengths of time, you are allowed to really contemplate your presence in your body. This gives you a stillness in which to begin to explore your mind/body connection. Focusing on your breath (discussed in Chapter 4) for these long periods of time can be extremely therapeutic, and, of course, relieve stress.

YOGIC WISDOM

If you suffer from anxiety, you are focusing on the future and have a hard time being in the present. You may experience heart palpitations and other physical symptoms. Restorative yoga helps ground you in the present, but don't overdo poses involving back bends, as they tend to increase anxiety.

Stress Reduction

Anxiety is a common psychological ill of our society, and creates a "hypervigilance" in the muscles of the body, leading them to become tightened and inflexible. Restorative yoga gives you an opportunity to really dissolve physical tension. But above all, it gives you an opportunity to "check in" with your body, to get in touch with it and gain control over your thoughts.

In our busy society, stress—which contributes to disease—is at an all-time high. It has been well documented that people are more frequently sick when they are stressed. We know that stress causes eating and related disorders, weight gain or loss, ulcers, and so much more. Stress is the cause of high blood pressure in about one-third of the population afflicted with related diseases. We also know that there are psychological pressures that cause anxiety and nervous disorders. It lessens well-being.

YOGIC WISDOM

Iyengar yoga teacher and sleep research scientist Roger Cole has done many studies on the benefits of restorative yoga. Roger is an Iyengar-trained yoga teacher who has been teaching since 1980. He is also an accomplished scientist who has studied sleep physiology at Stanford University, and has his doctorate in Health Psychology from the University of California. He is currently conducting sleep research, and has been able to explore the benefits of restorative yoga in his research as well. One of the most common effects of stress in our fast-paced, prescription-heavy era is troubled sleep. We need adequate, quality sleep now more than ever to counteract the stress of everyday life. When we can't sleep well, we drift further and further into an unhealthy state.

Dr. Herbert Benson, a cardiologist in Massachusetts who founded the Benson-Henry Institute for Mind Body Medicine at Massachusetts General Hospital, studied the idea of the "relaxation response"— the response of the body and mind when the mind consciously attempts to relax the body. This relaxation response explains how you can benefit from stress-reducing techniques such as restorative yoga. Restorative yoga works on the parasympathetic nervous system. Specific poses and sequences are set up to stimulate what needs to be stimulated, and calm down what needs calmed. It is much harder to calm down than it is to create tension or stimulation, but restorative yoga has techniques that effectively create this wonderful state of calm. In Part 2, you will discover all the poses and breathing techniques that you can use as tools to attain this state.

Yoga, as many people know it, is a form of physical activity. Unlike other forms of physical activity, there is a science to why certain poses work in some ways, and other poses work in other ways. This book hopes to provide you with an understanding of why that is, as it can be helpful to know why you are being told what poses to practice. It is how you can work best to get—keep—yourself healthy.

BALANCE OF ENERGIES

At the heart of restorative yoga is the balance of energies that flow throughout the body. When the body is in balance, a state of health is achieved. In the Eastern traditions, there are many ways of thinking about balancing these energies. Two of the most popular systems or philosophies that are applicable to how we practice restorative yoga are Ayurveda and chakras. Both are important to know as you try out the poses and sequences in Parts 2 and 3. Here is a brief overview of each system.

Ayurveda

Ayurveda, which means "science of life," is a body of Hindu knowledge and wisdom that has accumulated over many hundreds of years. Ayurvedic healing is an ancient practice and, much like traditional Chinese medicine, a holistic one. With the wisdom of Ayurvedic healing, one aims to address the person as a whole and eliminate the root cause of a person's illness, rather than just treating the symptoms by using the "Band-Aid" approach.

Like yoga, Ayurveda seeks to balance the body to instigate a state of health and well-being. In Ayurvedic wisdom, each individual is made up of a certain balance of doshas, or vital energies that make up the world. These doshas are called vata, pitta, and kapha, and each one has a unique quality. When these three doshas are in balance, the person is in a state of health. Disease occurs when the doshas shift out of balance. While everyone has all three doshas in their constitution—called a person's "doshic makeup"—one dosha will tend to be predominant. Understanding the doshas' qualities and evaluating your own doshic makeup can help you create an even more personalized restorative yoga practice. For example, if you have a dosha that is unbalanced, you can practice certain poses that will help you restore that balance. It's also helpful to understand that we all get out of balance, and even though our doshic makeup may feature a dosha that is more strongly present, we can treat imbalances if we understand the principles of Ayurveda.

Following is a more in-depth description of the doshas that make up your constitution. All three doshas can be brought into balance by restorative yoga practice. Each pose has either a stimulating, pacifying, or balancing aspect to it. You will find information that will indicate what to look for in each pose in Part 2.

- **Vata** (Air element): Vata is the more unstable dosha, and tends to go out of balance easily. When it's balanced, people are creative, but when it isn't balanced, they are erratic. Typical problems with this dosha are anxiety, irregular appetite, gas, bloating, constipation, and dry skin.

- **Pitta** (Fire and Water elements): Pitta is about digestion, heat, and transformation in the body. People with predominant Pitta doshas have sharp, intelligent minds. They tend to be workaholics and, if out of balance, can be judgmental and critical. These people tend to get ulcers and inflammation, bleed or bruise easily, and have high blood pressure.

- **Kapha** (Earth and Water elements): Kapha tends to be a stable and relaxed dosha. The body type of someone with a predominant Kapha tends to be heavier, but is steady, calm, and strong. They tend to be sweet, loving, and supportive people, but if out of balance they can be sluggish and lack motivation. Diabetes and depression can be common problems.

Applying Ayurvedic concepts to restorative yoga is very helpful, and you'll find icons signifying the poses that can help you balance your doshas in Part 2. Before you try to involve Ayurvedic wisdom in your restorative yoga practice, you need to determine your doshic makeup and learn more about the doshas in general. The best way is to see an Ayurvedic practitioner who can diagnose you, but you can also take the quiz found at *www .banyanbotanicals.com/constitutions/* to assess which dosha is most predominant in your makeup, so you can figure out which poses are best for you.

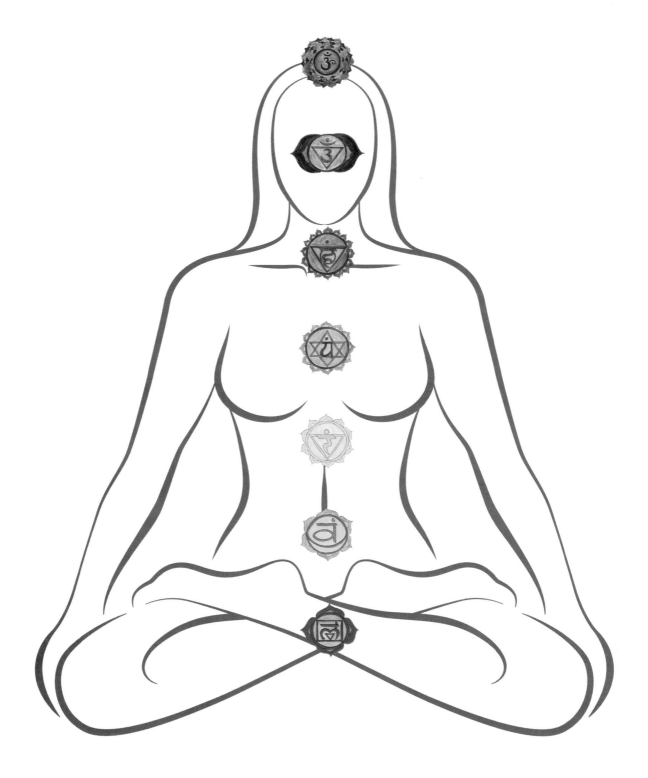

The Chakras

Chakras may seem esoteric, but when you understand the science behind them, you can learn how you can balance your energies. There are seven major chakras that are energy centers, or "wheels." As indicated in the previous image, they run up and down the midline of our bodies.

Each chakra is responsible for a certain aspect of body function, and also an aspect of your emotional state. Chakras spin like wheels as energy flows through them and, like any part of your body, they are subject to imbalances at any time. When a chakra is clear and energy runs through it properly, you will exhibit the best qualities that that particular chakra governs. When a chakra is not clear or somehow "stuck," energy will not be able to flow through it freely, and you will exhibit some imbalances relating to that chakra's qualities. Postures in yoga work to open, restore, and create a balanced flow of energy through each chakra. As you move to Part 2, you will see icons next to each pose to indicate which chakra or chakras that pose helps to open. You can use this information to help choose which postures you might need on a particular day, depending on how you feel.

Muladhara (Root Chakra)

The first chakra is the root chakra, which is located at the base the spine, deep in the pelvic floor. It is your "anchor," keeping you grounded physically and emotionally. The energy contained in the root chakra relates to the basics necessary for survival—food, sleep, and stability. If this chakra becomes imbalanced, you may be avoiding things you need to address, or you may start to develop fears. Hip opener poses are especially helpful in balancing this chakra.

Svadisthana (Pelvic Chakra)

The pelvic chakra is located in your pelvic chamber. It is related to your reproductive organs, and consequently, your desires. When things flow properly through this chakra, you not only have the potential to soothe yourself, you also are open to sensual pleasure. When this chakra is blocked, you may begin to develop attachments that are difficult to dislodge and that interrupt your life. Hip opener poses, as well as forward bends, can work to open this chakra and bring awareness concerning your deepest desires.

Manipura (Navel Chakra)

The navel chakra, better known as the "power center," is where your purpose in the outside world takes hold. This chakra rules your metabolism, and problems with this chakra may manifest as digestive issues. Your physical vitality and your individual power take root and flow through here. When this chakra is open and clear, you are able to carry out your individual purpose, whatever it may be. When this chakra is blocked, you may express aggressive ambition and selfishness in your pursuits. Twists are great for working through blockages here.

Anahata (Heart Chakra)

At the center of your chest is the heart chakra, the seat of your ability to love, be compassionate, and have faith. This chakra is associated with the lungs and the element of air, and is the "grand central station" for the flow of your emotional experiences. When blocked, you may radiate insecurity, despair, and loneliness instead of love. Back bends help to unblock this chakra.

Visuddha (Throat Chakra)

The throat chakra governs your speech and hearing. The endocrine glands are related to this chakra. This chakra's job is to ensure that you are able to communicate your truths and hear the truths of others, as well as converse freely and honestly. When you work with poses that open your throat area, such as Fish Pose, you help to stimulate this chakra.

Ajna (Third Eye Chakra)

Yogis believe there is a "third eye" that resides in the brain, about eyebrow level. This extra "eye" is connected to both your physical and emotional growth. When this chakra is open and your consciousness flows freely through it, you become in touch with your intuition, one of your most important guides. The pituitary gland is related to this chakra. Breathing practices (also known as *pranayama*) help to heal this chakra. You will learn more about these in Chapter 4.

Sahasrara (Crown Chakra)

The last chakra, the crown chakra, is considered the "crown" of the chakra system. It is the chakra that governs your highest state of development and enlightenment. It resides at the top of the head, and is understood to be the gateway to everything beyond our normal range of everyday experiences. Yogis believe that thought is the expression of this chakra. An overactive crown chakra causes you to feel as though you are part of an intellectual or spiritual elite. An underactive crown chakra distances you from your own spirituality, and may result in an unhealthy skepticism that blocks you from spiritual nourishment. Meditation is the best practice for clearing this chakra, and since restorative yoga poses are held for long periods of time, this practice gives you ample opportunity and space to practice meditation. If you're feeling muddle-minded, practicing meditation while in a restorative pose is a great way to combine these two practices and deeply restore your body and mind.

Restorative yoga is at the center of all the benefits mentioned in this chapter. It truly is a powerful tool to restoring and maintaining your body and its physical and energetic composition. Armed with the knowledge here, you can begin to go deeper into your practice by understanding what you need to have on hand to practice restorative yoga, how the poses work to restore you, and which ones will work best for you and your particular body composition and energetic makeup—which is always changing!

CHAPTER 3

GET READY TO PRACTICE RESTORATIVE YOGA

"Your hand opens and closes and opens and closes. If it were always a fist or always stretched open, you would be paralyzed. Your deepest presence is in every small contracting and expanding, the two as beautifully balanced and coordinated as bird wings."

—Rumi, thirteenth-century poet and Sufi mystic

So now that you know what restorative yoga is and how it can help you find balance both physically and emotionally, what exactly do you need to have on hand to practice restorative yoga? Restorative yoga depends on a variety of props to ensure that you feel supported and comfortable, and in this chapter you'll learn what you need and how to use it. In addition, you'll need to make sure that you have a physical space to practice where you feel comfortable and safe. You'll also learn how to prepare your space for restorative yoga. After all, it's difficult to clear your mind and stretch your body if you're wondering if someone's going to barge in, or if a ringing cell phone constantly disturbs your peace. So let's take a look at what you need to set yourself up for restorative yoga.

SETTING UP THE SPACE

When setting up a space for your restorative yoga practice, think about one word: comfort. You will need to create a space that will help you truly relax. Here are some key points to remember when setting up the space:

- First, make sure the space you are in is as dark as possible, as bright light will keep you too stimulated.

- Minimize noise. Make sure your space is as free from outside noise as possible. Relaxing music is fine, but even with the most relaxing music, remember that the thoughts that come while listening can sometimes keep you from truly being able to let go. Make sure you're in a space where nothing can distract you.

- The temperature of the room should be warm, and you should dress warmly. Have extra layers available. If you are cold, you cannot relax. Your body temperature will drop as you relax, so it's a good idea to plan ahead.

- Take off your watch. The watch represents your attachments to time, so in order to truly let go, don't wear a watch when you practice. Instead, use a timer with a pleasant-sounding chime to keep track of how long you are in each pose.

As you set up your space, keep in mind that it may not always be possible to be completely free from all distractions, but do the best you can to leave the outside world behind. Shut off your phone, and take the time you need. In the end, it will make you a healthier, more productive person.

PROPS

Restorative yoga is a prop-heavy practice. The props are essential to the practice because they help your body fully relax into the positions so you can truly "let go." Certain props are used more than others, and depending on the issue, you may not need specific ones. Blankets are probably the most versatile—and most used—of all props because you can roll them or fold them, adjusting them to achieve the desired effect of either less opening or more opening, less support or more support. Following is a list of the most common restorative yoga props that you want to have on hand:

Blocks

You want to make sure that you have a minimum of two blocks on hand before starting restorative yoga. Blocks can be made of cork, wood, or foam. I recommend purchasing ones made of dense foam. Dense foam blocks are sturdier than the other kinds, and if used directly on the body, are softer than cork or wood. Blocks are great because they can prop your body up in areas that need support, are very easy to work with, and don't take up a lot of space. I recommend using blocks that measure 4" × 6" × 9".

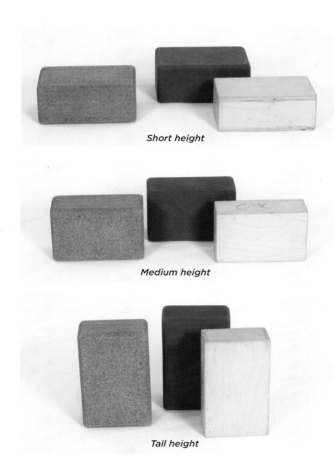

Short height

Medium height

Tall height

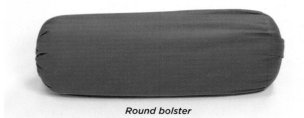

Round bolster

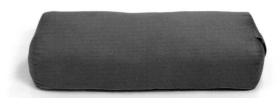

Flat bolster

(For each block, there are three standard heights: short, medium, and tall. In my practice, I refer to these as the "baby bear," "mama bear," and "papa bear," but I've given you the more standard height descriptors throughout.)

Bolsters

A bolster is the main prop of restorative yoga that you rest on while in your pose. In a perfect situation, you would have a flat and a round bolster for your practice, but you can create bolsters out of blankets if need be. Flat bolsters are approximately 8" × 27" × 32.5", and round bolsters are approximately 9" × 26" × 34.5". If you are looking to recreate them with blankets, these measurements are important. These two bolsters can be used interchangeably throughout the poses and sequences. Use whatever feels comfortable as you practice.

Blankets

Blankets provide extra cushioning and warmth during the practice of restorative yoga. Traditional yoga blankets are either made of wool, or are Mexican-style blankets that are either cotton or a cotton/wool blend. You want to use a blanket that's around 75" × 52" in size, so keep that in mind if using a blanket from your home.

The blanket's added weight will help you to relax while in the poses. You can also use a blanket to create a swaddling effect, which will subconsciously remind you of when you were a baby and felt cared for, automatically creating a sense of relaxation. Blankets can also be used to provide full or partial support, or, as previously mentioned, they can be layered to create a bolster. Since there are many ways that you can work with a blanket, it's important for you to know the many ways they can be manipulated and used. Here are some of the key folds that are referred to in the Poses and Sequences in Parts 2 and 3:

Open Fold: Keep the blanket open to use as extra cushioning on the floor, or for draping over your body.

Half Fold: Fold the blanket in half lengthwise or widthwise to provide extra cushioning, as your yoga mat may not make the floor as soft as you would like it to be.

Oblong Fold: Beginning with the Half Fold, fold the blanket in half lengthwise and again in half lengthwise.

Square Fold: This is the basic shape that most of the following folds typically start with. Fold the blanket in half from the short side, then fold again two more times. "WWW" is a great way to remember how to make this fold (fold "Width, by Width, by Width").

Small Square: Beginning with the Square Fold, fold the blanket in half widthwise.

Short Roll: Beginning with the Square Fold, roll the blanket with the fringe or open side on either right or left.

Long Roll: Beginning with the Square Fold, roll the blanket with the fringe or open side facing you. Roll fringe in toward the smooth side.

Accordion: Beginning with the long side of the Square Fold, fold the blanket in quarters or thirds, accordion style.

Head Rest Fold: Beginning with the Square Fold, fold blanket almost in half widthwise, so the edges are staggered by about 6 inches. To make this fold even more supportive, sometimes you can fold it in from the sides or roll it up a little bit at the neck to support the seventh cervical vertebra.

Rectangle Fold: Beginning with the Square Fold, fold the blanket in half lengthwise.

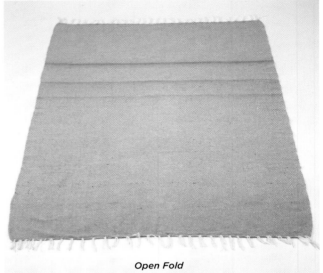

Open Fold

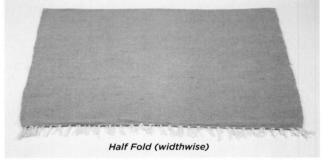

Half Fold (widthwise)

Oblong Fold

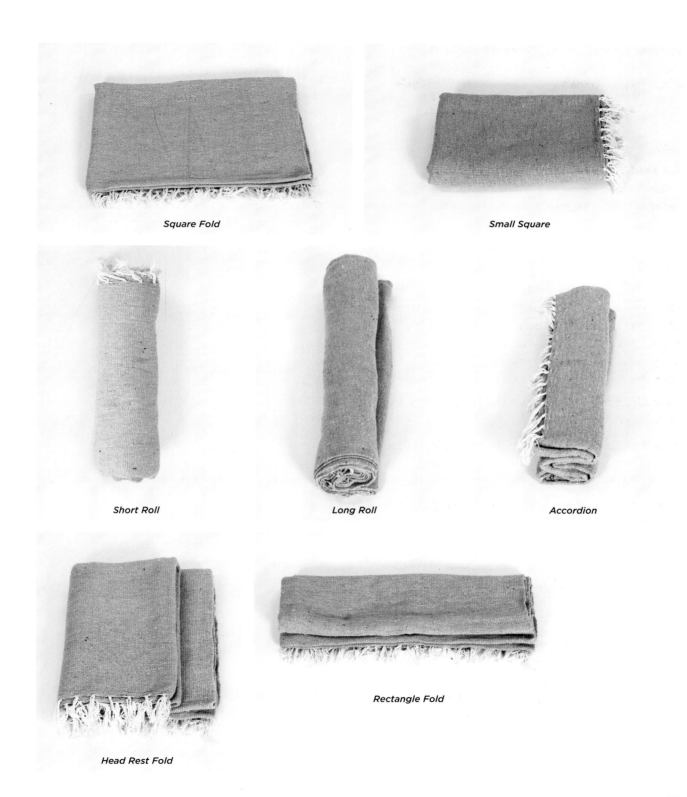

Square Fold

Small Square

Short Roll

Long Roll

Accordion

Head Rest Fold

Rectangle Fold

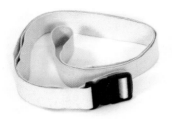

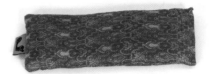

Strap

Straps are commonly used in yoga to lengthen your body's span. For example, if you can't reach your feet with your hands, the strap enables you to reach. You can also use them as a tool to help you get a proper stretch. In restorative yoga, they are also used for creating stability during rest. This stability helps you rest in a stretch without effort, making a strap an essential restorative yoga prop. A 10-inch strap belt will give you the most options. I like the quick-release belts the best, since they offer the fastest way to get in and out of them. You can use any kind you have, though, and could even use an old tie if you don't have a chance to purchase a proper yoga strap.

Chair

Chairs are used for many of the shapes that you hold in restorative yoga. A regular folding chair or specialized backless yoga chair is the best type of chair to use, because they have a flat seat. Backless chairs are a little easier to use than regular folding chairs, and can be bought from many yoga supply sources. If you use a folding chair, make sure it feels sturdy. It's hard to relax if your chair does not feel supportive. In some cases, a chair can be used instead of a bolster or a wall.

Sandbag

Sandbags are used in restorative yoga for "grounding," which means that they are placed on specific parts of the body to add weight to that area. Grounding is an important part of the practice; it helps deepen the sense of support that opens up relaxation and stimulates healing. If you don't want to purchase yoga-specific sandbags, a 10-pound bag of rice wrapped in a pillowcase works just as well.

Eye Bag/Eye Pillow

Eye bags and eye pillows are good additions to any restorative yoga pose, as they help to relax the eyes and block out light. Keep them handy to deepen the sense of relaxation you feel as you stay in the pose, especially during Savasana, the corpse pose (see Chapter 5). It's traditionally done at the end of practice to seal in all the previous poses and allow your body to really absorb the effect of the practice.

Headwrap

A traditional yoga headwrap looks like an ACE bandage. It is wrapped around the head tightly to create a calming pressure, which induces a state of relaxation. Headwraps are mainly used in the postures that target headaches and head tension, but they are great to use anytime. You can purchase a proper headwrap online from the Iyengar Institute (*https://iynaus.org/store/store/props*).

Yoga Mat

For any posture where you sit or lie down, a yoga mat will come in handy. It provides extra cushioning from the hard floor if you are practicing on one. For standing postures or those that are more complicated and involve chairs, a yoga mat can prevent slipping. Yoga mats also provide a clean space for you to practice. If you do not have a yoga mat, you can use a large towel or a blanket.

Wall

Several poses in this book require a wall—in fact, it is a main source of support in restorative yoga. The good news is that there are walls everywhere you go, and you don't need to purchase them! You may want to clear a wall space in your home specifically for the purpose of restorative yoga. That way, when you use that particular wall again and again, you'll really feel "at home" when you return to it.

Use What Works

Many poses can be set up with minimal props, and you may even be able to use what you have at home to engage in this practice without breaking the bank buying new materials. Couch cushions and pillows, for example, make great bolsters, and a necktie works well as a yoga strap. Books can be your "blocks," a washcloth can work as your "eye pillow," and regular home blankets and towels can be your

extra "blankets." You don't need to feel that you have to purchase all the yoga props there are on the market. But don't skimp: One truth when it comes to props is the more the merrier! Always feel free to add additional props as needed. You can truly never have enough. The name of the game is *comfort*, and when you are comfortable you can truly heal.

Setting up a space that you return to again and again at home is a great way to commit to the practice. Consider leaving the props handy in the space in case you are so tired that the thought of setting up for more complicated postures discourages you from practicing. Keep in mind that restorative yoga is a practice that can be done by everybody. Whether you are physically fit or not, energized or fatigued, adjusted or stressed, restorative yoga is a powerful tool that will help you connect to your body. Whether you have props or not, are traveling or at home, you can improvise what you need to do these poses.

So, now that you've learned how to set up the key elements of your practice, it's time to get started!

YOGIC WISDOM

Here are some suggested links to online sources of yoga props. I recommend any of these sources. All of them provide what you need at affordable prices:

- *www.innerspaceyoga.net*
- *www.toolsforyoga.net*
- *www.yogamoves.net*
- *www.huggermugger.com*
- *www.yogadirect.com*
- *www.amazon.com*
- *www.myzenhome.com*
- *www.yogalifestyle.com*

PART 2

GETTING STARTED

"Our bodies are apt to be our autobiographies."
—Frank Gelett Burgess, American artist, art critic, poet, author, and humorist

Here is where it all begins: the poses. This part of the book contains all the restorative yoga poses you need to build a full restorative yoga practice. The poses are broken up into categories: warm-ups, back bends, twists, forward bends, and inversions. Warm-ups help you to settle in; back bends energize by opening the front body; twists tone your organs by wringing out toxins in the body; forward bends calm and soothe by closing the front body in a position of surrender; and inversions help bring the body's total systems into balance. You'll also find a chapter that gives you detailed information on various breathing techniques and visualizations that can help you "let go" as you practice the poses found here and seal in the practice and its benefits.

Throughout Parts 2 and 3, you'll also find sidebars focusing on the Yoga Sutras of Patanjali, a compilation of 196 "threads of thought" that offer wisdom derived from the practice of yoga. I often find that once students begin to find a deeper connection to their inner self through the physical practice of yoga, they begin to look for philosophy to support their personal growth. These "threads of thought" will help to support your practice.

Keep in mind that while the breathing exercises and poses found in this part are not aerobically demanding, they will energize you all the same. So get ready to be restored and renewed. All you need to do is gather your props, set yourself up, and relax.

CHAPTER 4

BREATHING AND VISUALIZATIONS

"What lies behind you and what lies in front of you, pales in comparison to what lies inside of you."

—Ralph Waldo Emerson, American essayist and poet

Pranayama, usually translated to mean "breath control," is one of the "eight limbs of yoga" according to Patanjali. Breathing techniques have their own power to heal our bodies by connecting us to our breath, which creates physiological and psychological changes that ultimately restore balance in the body and mind. These practices are just as—if not more important—than the postures in yoga.

In this chapter, you'll find standard breathing techniques that are taught in yoga. Learning how to do these techniques and when to apply them will help your restorative yoga practice become that much more effective. These techniques can be practiced while seated or lying down, and many can be done while in your restorative poses to help you settle in and quiet the mind. Return to these practices often so that they become second nature to you, and you'll be able to incorporate them into your yoga practice when you most need them.

Note: Pranayama, if practiced incorrectly, can have damaging effects as well. The techniques that I have shared with you are ones that are simple to practice on your own without the guidance of a certified teacher at your side.

CENTERING

One of the first—and most important—things to do when beginning a restorative yoga practice is centering. Centering gives you an opportunity to become more focused on what you are doing in the here and now. Just as it sounds, you get connected to your "center." When you center, you become more present and clear about what you are feeling throughout your body. For example, you'll be able to identify where you feel pain, where you feel energy, and so forth. Arming yourself with this information will help you see what areas are calling out for attention, so you can use the poses and sequences in Parts 2 and 3 to design your own personal restorative yoga practice. Throughout this chapter, you will learn a few specific techniques that utilize the breath to help create a sense of calm in your body. To begin, here is a centering exercise to help you get started.

CENTERING EXERCISE

As you practice this breathing exercise, notice what is happening in your body. Scan for any discomfort. When focusing on the breath, you become more present in your body. As you become more present, it becomes more about the here and now, and less about what happened in the past or what is going to happen in the future. When you are present you can focus on what really is going on for you in that moment.

1. Come to a comfortable seated position either in a chair or on the floor.

2. If you sit on a chair, bring yourself toward the front of the chair, so your sitting bones (literally the bones that are covered by the flesh of your buttocks) are touching the chair and you are not leaning back. Your spine should be lengthened. If you sit on the floor, you may need to raise your seat on a blanket or a block so your hips are above your knees. If your hips are already above your knees, you don't need to raise your seat. If it's difficult to keep the spine upright, you can sit against a wall.

3. Use your breath as a point of focus. As you inhale, follow the breath in through your nostrils; as you exhale, follow the breath out your nostrils. Initially you may just focus on the simple entry and exit point of the breath. If you are comfortable closing your eyes, it can help keep you more focused on this task. You may also choose to look down with a soft gaze.

4. As you continue to breathe, start to connect the breath with the lungs and the diaphragm by following the path of air as it is drawn into the lungs. The full and complete breath is ultimately the goal. Take as deep an inhalation as feels comfortable, and as deep an exhalation as feels comfortable. You may notice some discomfort emotionally as you begin this practice. If you start to feel anxious, shorten your inhalation and focus on the deep exhalation. Try to stay with this practice for five full minutes.

YOGIC WISDOM

To understand what really ails you, you have to be quiet and listen. Sometimes performing a preliminary informational "self-interview" can help pinpoint your pain even further. Here is a list of questions you can ask yourself:

- *What hurts?*
- *How did it happen?*
- *How long have I had the pain?*
- *What time of day or when does it hurt me the most?*
- *Have I received any professional opinions on my situation? What were they?*

Using a journal, write down your answers. Read them back to yourself. What do you understand about your pain? Think about your answers as you develop your practice—what kinds of poses do you think you would benefit from most?

BREATHING EXERCISES

We now know scientifically that controlling the breath helps to calm the mind. It is even believed to contribute to a longer life. Typically, when you are able to control your breath, you feel more at harmony with your body and mind, have less anxiety, and can even stabilize high blood pressure. Overall, you will feel more focused, clear, and happy in your daily life. As you prepare to practice these breathing exercises, know that your eyes can be closed, but if you are not comfortable closing your eyes, look down slightly and try to soften your gaze.

APA JAPA BREATH

Apa Japa means "breath awareness." The purpose of this breathing technique is to become aware of your body by becoming aware of your breath. It is a great tool for centering, and becoming attuned to any tension and where you are holding it. Use it prior to practicing yoga or during your restorative poses to settle in.

1. Lie down or come to a comfortable seated position either in a chair or on the floor. Feel free to use a blanket under your bottom for comfort and/or sit against a wall for back support. Once you are comfortable, close your eyes and direct your attention inward.

2. Do not try to change anything, just bring your awareness to your breath. Drawing your attention to your breath will naturally cause you to change your breathing pattern, but try to avoid it. This is the challenge of the technique. Just let your breath be natural.

3. Focus on the length of your inhalation and the length of your exhalation.

4. Notice where you feel your breath. Notice it coming in through the nostrils and into your lungs. Feel the breath as it travels into your lungs and fills your lungs. Notice the expansion and contraction of your ribs as you breathe in and out.

5. Keep breathing like this for at least two minutes.

DIAPHRAGMATIC BREATH

This breathing technique helps you to breathe "bigger." It helps you train the muscles in your abdomen and diaphragm to open up and take in more breath. Note that you may do this pose seated or lying down, but you may feel that you can better connect to this while lying down.

1. Lie down or come to a comfortable seated position either in a chair or on the floor. Once you are comfortable, place one hand on your abdomen and one hand on your chest.

2. Breathe into your abdomen using your diaphragm, and feel the hand rise as it fills and feel it lower as you exhale.

3. Follow this movement and notice where your breath is traveling.

4. See if you can bring the breath into the abdomen so your breath is more expansive.

BREATH WITH PAUSE

In this breathing technique, you retain the breath (known as kumbhaka) in order to sharpen your awareness. This sense of stillness you search out in this breathing technique is the beginning of meditation practice—the practice of finding calmness and equanimity with the self.

1. Lie down or come to a comfortable seated position either in a chair or on the floor. Once you are comfortable, take a full diaphragmatic breath into your abdomen, then pause immediately after your inhalation, until you feel you need to exhale.

2. Exhale and pause immediately after your exhalation, until you feel you need to inhale again.

3. Practice for a minimum of two minutes.

> **YOGIC WISDOM**
>
> *Do not hold the breath for long pauses; just hold long enough give yourself an opportunity to notice the space between the breaths.*

UJJAII BREATH

This breathing technique has been shown to slow the synapses of the brain down. In yoga, it is also known as "victorious breath." I tell students that they should sound like Darth Vader breathing or ocean waves along the shore as they do it. This technique is often used in active styles of yoga because the constriction of the throat needed to make this breath happen warms your body from the inside out.

OPTION 1

1. Come to a comfortable seated position either in a chair or on the floor so that your chin doesn't restrict your throat by causing it to be too open or too closed. Support yourself with any props you need for comfort. Once you are comfortable, practice constricting your throat (technically the glottis). Place your hand in front of your open mouth and breathe out, as if fogging a pair of glasses. Notice that the breath is warm.

2. The hardest part is breathing in. Try to constrict the throat as you breathe in.

3. After you have practiced a bit with the mouth open, try to explore this with the mouth closed. Just breathe in and out of your nostrils while constricting the throat for about one minute.

YOGIC WISDOM

This breath can be used as a relaxation technique for many different issues. It can be used to help ease insomnia, stress, and as a technique to calm down before speaking out of turn. It helps in almost any tense situation to center you and help you relax. The only time this breath is not recommended is during the Savasana poses, when the throat should be relaxed.

OPTION 2

1. Lie down or come to a comfortable seated position either in a chair or on the floor. Once you are comfortable, inhale for the count of two and exhale for the count of four.

2. Continue to breathe to this count. After about thirty seconds, increase the count: Inhale for a count of three and exhale for a count of six, and so on.

3. Find a comfortable count at which to continue—you don't want to feel any anxiety. This breath should help you to feel calm. Practice for five minutes, if possible.

YOGIC WISDOM

This breathing exercise is great for calming the mind and the sympathetic nervous system (SNS), which is the part of your body that commands your fight-or-flight response. When you practice this exercise, the vagus nerve, which runs down the neck through your diaphragm, sends a message to your brain to activate your parasympathetic nervous system (PSNS), which is responsible for the "rest and digest" or "feed and breed" responses that are triggered when relaxation is achieved. The sympathetic nervous system creates cortisol in your system as a result of the fight-or-flight activation. When you practice this exercise, the parasympathetic system works to lower the cortisol that wreaks havoc on your system.

ALTERNATE NOSTRIL BREATHING

Also known as Nadi Shodana, this technique helps to create balance between the right and the left sides of the brain. In yogic thought, the right side is believed to be the masculine side, which harnesses the sun energy known as *Ha* and the left side is believed to be the feminine side, which harnesses the moon energy known as *Tha*. (Hence the term *Hatha* yoga.) When it comes to breathing, every 88 minutes, either our left or right nostril is dominant. Alternate nostril breathing tricks the brain so it does not know which nostril should be dominant, allowing the breath to flow more evenly through each nostril. When you use this technique, your brain and the nervous system become balanced and you can more easily move into a state of meditation.

1. Come to a comfortable seated position either in a chair or on the floor. Once you are comfortable, rest your left hand on your left leg.

2. Using your right hand, bring your peace fingers (pointer and middle finger) to your third eye (between your eyebrows) or fold them into the heel of your hand.

3. Gently place your ring finger and thumb on either side of your nose, where the hard cartilage and the soft cartilage meet. Exhale and inhale through both nostrils. After inhaling, gently pinch your nose to close off your nostrils. Release the pressure on the left side only, so that the right nostril is blocked, and exhale on the left.

4. Inhale on the left, then hold the left nostril and exhale on the right.

5. Inhale on the right, hold the right nostril, and then exhale on the left.

6. Continue to practice this for at least six rounds. (A round includes an inhale holding and an exhale holding on both sides.)

7. When the exercise is complete, bring both hands to rest on your legs and breathe regularly.

YOGIC WISDOM

We have three main nadis, or energy channels, throughout our bodies. The central channel is called Sahshumna nadi, and the energy runs from the base of the spine up to the crown of the head. The two other nadis are Ida and Pingala, which crisscross through the central nadi. Ida is considered the "female" channel, and Pingala the "male" channel, as their complementary qualities are likened to yin/yang, dark/light, or sun/moon. Ida starts on the left, and Pingala starts on the right.

SITALI BREATH

Sitali Breath is a cooling breathing technique. The best way to understand this is to look at a dog. Dogs pant, using their tongues to cool themselves down. Think of your tongue as a straw and curl the sides of your tongue inward to do this breath. Not everyone is able to curl their tongue, so if you cannot, just let the tongue hang out of your mouth, like a dog.

1. Come to a comfortable seated position, either in a chair or on the floor. Once you are comfortable, stick your tongue out of your mouth, either curled like a straw or flat.

2. Inhale, allowing the air to travel up the tongue. After you inhale, bring your tongue back into your mouth, then close your mouth and exhale through your nose. You will feel how cooling it is.

3. Practice this breath anytime you need to cool yourself down. You can practice this breathing technique for one to two minutes at a time.

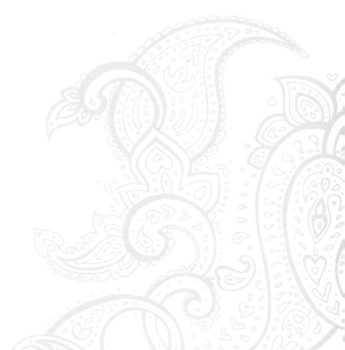

VISUALIZATIONS/ MANTRA MEDITATIONS

The mind can be difficult to harness, as we often have many thoughts going on at one time. The following visualization techniques and mantra meditations will help quiet your mind.

CLOUD

Clouds are a wonderful visual aid for meditation, as everyone can bring the image of a cloud to their mind somewhat easily. Clouds can float by quickly or slowly, and so can your thoughts. The more space you have between your thoughts, the easier it will be for your mind to achieve quietude.

1. Lie down or come to a comfortable seated position either in a chair or on the floor. Feel free to use a blanket under your bottom for comfort and/or sit against a wall for back support. Once you are comfortable, close your eyes and direct your attention inward.

2. As you are settling in, you may notice the thoughts that come to the forefront of your mind. Sometimes we have a lot of thoughts bombarding us, other days it's not as bad, but either way, we are looking to find the space between the thoughts. To do this, as each thought comes, imagine placing it on a cloud, and watch it drift past.

3. As you practice this visualization exercise regularly, you will begin to find that your thoughts have more space between them, and you don't have to place as many on clouds.

4. Try to practice this visualization technique for five minutes to begin with, and gradually build up to a half an hour.

STRAW

When focusing your attention on the breath, it can be helpful to use a visualization to help you connect even deeper. It's easy to visualize your spine as a straw, and very helpful to visualize your breath like liquid traveling up that straw as you sip, and the liquid pooling back in the bottom of the glass as you let go.

1. Lie down or come to a comfortable seated position either in a chair or on the floor. Feel free to use a blanket under your bottom for comfort and/or sit against a wall for back support. Once you are comfortable, close your eyes and direct your attention inward.

2. Visualize that you are sitting in a pool of white light.

3. Visualize your spine as a straw. As you inhale, visualize that you are sipping the white light at the base of your spine up the straw of your spine. As you exhale, let the light flow back down the straw of your spine.

4. Try to do this visualization technique for five minutes, and gradually build up to a half an hour.

WHITE LIGHT

White light is considered a cleansing, healing light. Filling yourself with this light is a helpful way to access this healing energy. Using this visualization, you can direct your breath to areas of the body that are in need of healing. Whether there is a specific spot in your body that is painful or whether you are healing from cancer, this is an incredibly beneficial tool. You will find this visualization incorporated in the cancer sequence (see Part 3) and cancer cells are specifically mentioned here, but feel free to use it anywhere or anytime you feel inclined.

1. Lie down or come to a comfortable seated position either in a chair or on the floor. Feel free to use a blanket under your bottom for comfort and/or sit against a wall for back support. Once you are comfortable, close your eyes and direct your attention inward.

2. Visualize where the cancer cells/pains are in your body.

3. See the white light enveloping the cancer cells/pains and eradicating any trace of them.

4. Follow the white light as it travels around, eradicating any cancer cells/pains it finds, enveloping them with the light and moving on to the next spot.

5. Continue to do this until you feel you have gotten to every possible cancer cell/pain that is in your body.

6. Try to do this visualization technique for five minutes, and gradually build up to a half an hour.

HUM SAH MANTRA MEDITATION

Mantra meditation can be very powerful, as it is a way to tether your mind by giving it something neutral to focus on. The Hum Sah mantra means "I am that," and it is a wonderful way of connecting you with everything, helping you avoid a sense of conflict from your little self and the bigger picture around you. Hum Sah sounds like the noise your breath makes when you inhale and exhale, but you are not meant to say it out loud, just hear it in your mind.

1. Lie down or come to a comfortable seated position either in a chair or on the floor. Feel free to use a blanket under your bottom for comfort and/or sit against a wall for back support. Once you are comfortable, close your eyes and direct your attention inward.

2. As you inhale say silently to yourself "hum," and as you exhale, silently say "sah."

3. You can also visualize the breath as light going up and down the spine at the same time.

4. Try to do this meditation technique for five minutes, and gradually build up to a half an hour.

WORD MEDITATION

Mantras do not need to be words in another language. Feel free to use a word of your choosing, and repeat that for your mantra. It may be associated with something you are working on bringing more of into your life. Popular words to choose are "love" or "peace," but use whatever word resonates with you. This is a nice, relaxed way to explore using a mantra.

1. Lie down or come to a comfortable seated position either in a chair or on the floor. Feel free to use a blanket under your bottom for comfort and/or sit against a wall for back support. Once you are comfortable, close your eyes and direct your attention inward.

2. As you inhale, say to yourself your word, and as you exhale, repeat the word.

3. Try to do this meditation technique for five minutes, and gradually build up to a half an hour.

VARIATION

As an alternative to this meditation, you may just repeat your chosen word over and over again without timing it to the rhythm of your breath. For example, just keep repeating "peace, peace, peace, peace . . . ." You can visualize what it means to have this in your life as you repeat the word. Feel it in your body.

YOGA NIDRA

True Yoga Nidra is a very detailed, methodical practice that allows you to look at your body, part by part, as you move deeper into a state of relaxation called yogic sleep. This particular process is really just Yoga Nidra in name alone, as it is not meant to take you into a yogic sleep, but just to deepen your state of relaxation. In this visualization, your attention is drawn briefly to each part of your body, and you move on to the next spot swiftly. Feel free to record yourself reading this aloud, and listen to the recording instead of trying to remember all of this. You will find it hard to relax if you have to really think about it.

1. To practice this technique it is best to lie down. Make sure you are comfortable with any props that you need to support you. Once you are comfortable, close your eyes and direct your attention inward.

2. Begin by directing your attention to your feet. Relax your feet and your toes, then move your attention up your legs. Relax your calves, your shins, your knees, your thighs, and your buttocks. Relax your lower back, your abdomen, your chest, then your shoulders. Relax your arms, then relax your fingers. Feel your whole arm relax, and allow that relaxation to travel back up your arm to your relaxed shoulders, then relax your neck and all the muscles in your face. Relax your scalp, and feel your whole body settle deeper into the floor, then let go of any remaining tension.

3. Systematically go through each body part again and become more specific. For example, when you get to your hands, relax your right pinky, ring finger, middle finger, index finger, and thumb. Then relax your left pinky, ring finger, middle finger, index finger, and thumb.

4. A true session of Yoga Nidra can take more than an hour, but you should try this variation for only a few minutes, and slowly work up to longer sessions.

CHAPTER 5

THE POSES

*"Yoga is the perfect opportunity to be curious
about who you are."*

—Jason Crandell, American yoga teacher

Now that you know how to center yourself and are familiar with the breathing and meditative exercises that will help prepare you for restorative yoga, it's time to take a look at the variety of restorative yoga poses that will help you feel at ease in your body, recover from illness or physical injury, and gain a sense of balance and well-being. Keep in mind that there is no one correct way to go about choosing the restorative yoga poses from this chapter. You can practice one pose at a time, or mix and match based on what intuitively seems right for your body on any given day. You may notice that a pose creates feelings for you on a physical or emotional level. Pay attention to those feelings. Think about where they might be coming from. It's helpful to practice with this level of awareness, as it will help your practice come from a more intuitive place. Ultimately, you have the innate wisdom to heal yourself, if you pay attention. The more you practice these poses, the more you will find what resonates with you and helps you to restore some balance in your body where you most need it. To help you with this, Part 3 takes the poses that you'll learn here and puts them into sequences that will help you go further to address specific issues you may have—whether they be physical or emotional.

As you try these poses, remember that each person's body is different, and some poses will work better for you than others. For example, some poses may prove to be especially challenging and difficult to get into, depending on your level of fitness and flexibility. To that end, there are variations offered to help you find comfort in each pose. Spend some time figuring out what works best for you with each pose: Give yourself the freedom to experiment, and don't rush. Remember, you want to feel supported and comfortable so that you can fully relax. You will feel most relaxed when you are supported well, which may simply mean that you should add an extra blanket or block. Play around until you feel right, right where you are.

WHAT TO LOOK FOR

Throughout this chapter, you will see a set of symbols beside each pose. One set refers to chakras, which, as discussed in Chapter 2, are energy centers in the body that are stimulated by yoga postures. The following chakra icons are used to indicate which chakra(s) each pose activates:

- Muladhara (Root Chakra):

- Svadisthana (Pelvic Chakra):

- Manipura (Navel Chakra):

- Anahata (Heart Chakra):

- Visuddha (Throat Chakra):

- Ajna (Third Eye Chakra):

- Sahasrara (Crown Chakra):

The other set of symbols found next to each pose refers to the doshas, which were also discussed in Chapter 2. For each pose, you will see a V (for Vata), P (for Pitta), or a K (for Kapha) with a =, +, or – sign next to it. The = means a pose is balancing, the + means it increases the dosha, and the – means it decreases the dosha. This information can be beneficial in choosing poses to practice, depending on your particular doshic imbalance. Keep in mind that all doshic makeups, no matter what their imbalances, can benefit from poses that balance Vata, as Vata is the dosha responsible for movement. Sometimes you need to increase it, and sometimes you need to decrease it.

GENERAL RESTORATIVE YOGA POSE TIPS

Before you begin practicing the poses in this chapter, it's important that you have a clear picture of who you are within the context of your restorative yoga practice—what your physical limitations are, what you may need to pay attention to physically and emotionally at any given time, where you are seeing results and want to continue doing, and vice versa. Frequently rereading these tips as you progress will help you check in with yourself to make sure you're getting the most out of your restorative yoga practice.

- Never hold a position that is uncomfortable to the point of pain. Sensation is okay; pain is not.

- Discomfort, either physical or emotional, is sometimes a normal part of the practice.

- Your breath should flow smoothly.

- Allow yourself to be held up and supported by your props. Do not try to put in too much effort in any way.

- Notice that at first a pose may feel difficult, but it gets easier to be in the pose with time.

- Give yourself time to practice. Most poses should be held for a minimum of five minutes.

- Remember that quiet, warm, dark environments are important for a true sense of relaxation to set in.

- Stay comfortable in the poses. Covering yourself with a blanket during a pose is a great way to increase a sense of relaxation. The added weight adds a little extra warmth as well as a sense of security. Eye pillows can be placed over your eyes for an added sense of relaxation as well. Keep extra blankets and eye pillows within reach around you for easy access after you set up the pose. Even if eye pillows or blankets are not specifically listed for a pose, feel free to add them.

- Before moving on to sequences, make sure you know the How Tos of each individual pose thoroughly.

- Take time to set up the poses. Make adjustments so that you can be comfortable while practicing, as comfort is of the utmost importance. Props can be interchanged: an oblong or rectangular bolster substituted for a round bolster, a different fold or roll of blanket, and even using a blanket instead of a bolster. Make the pose and props work for your body.

- As we discussed in Chapter 3, be sure to take off your watch, but use a timer so you don't have to think about the time. If possible, choose a sound on your timer that is peaceful, not jarring.

It doesn't matter who you are, whether you're overweight, underweight, or have a specific ailment. Whoever you are, wherever you are in your life, you can practice these restorative yoga poses with comfort and ease. Keep in mind that you want to be as comfortable as possible when practicing the poses, and that some may provide extra cushioning and support, some less. Feel free to add additional props or remove some if that's what you need to do to feel comfortable and at ease.

> ### THREADS OF THOUGHT
>
> **Sthira sukham asanam**
>
> *Keep your yoga postures stable (sthira) yet light (sukham).*

WARM-UPS

You may be thinking, "Warm-ups in restorative yoga? Isn't restorative yoga relaxing enough?" The fact is that warm-up stretches prepare the body to really let go, which is the goal of restorative yoga. With a relaxed body, you set yourself up mentally and physically to really settle into the poses. These warm-up poses set you up by helping you connect with your breath and your surroundings, including the props that you will be using later. Take your time in each pose, and slowly become aware of your breath and what's underneath and around you. Are you settling in? Beginning to relax? Choose from the following poses to warm up, focusing on poses that address problem areas in your body where you might need a little extra loosening. You only need to do a few of these stretches to set yourself up for practice.

EXTENDED HAND TO FOOT POSE, SUPINE

Chakras Benefited:

Doshic Balance: K+, P+, V=

This pose helps open and stretch your back, legs, and hips. It can be done without the wall, and without a blanket or block as well. In a more active class you would balance on one leg to hold this pose, but it's much easier to achieve when you're lying down!

YOU NEED:
- Mat
- Wall (optional)
- Blanket (Head Rest Fold) (optional)
- Strap
- Block (optional)

WHAT TO DO

1. Lie on your back with your legs straight. If desired, press your feet against a wall for stability. Place a Head Rest Fold blanket under your head if you need the support. If it's uncomfortable on your back, you can bend the leg keeping the foot on the floor on the side that is not being held by the strap.

2. Holding one end of the strap in each hand, hug one knee into your chest and place the arch of your foot in the strap to make a loop. Straighten your leg until it's perpendicular to the floor. Stay in this position for two minutes for the stretch to really be effective, but if you can't, try to hold it for at least one minute on each side.

3. Now move both ends of the strap into the hand on the same side as the leg that is extended upright. At this point you may place a block next to your leg right by your hip for support, if desired. Open the leg out to the side. Hold this pose for a minimum of one minute.

4. Now bring the leg back upright, and switch the strap ends to the opposite hand. Keeping tension on the strap, swing your leg over to the opposite side. Feel free to place a block under your foot for support if necessary. You should hold this position where you feel the stretch the most; you may not even have to bring the foot anywhere near the floor or block. Hold for a minimum of one minute.

5. Repeat this pose with the other leg.

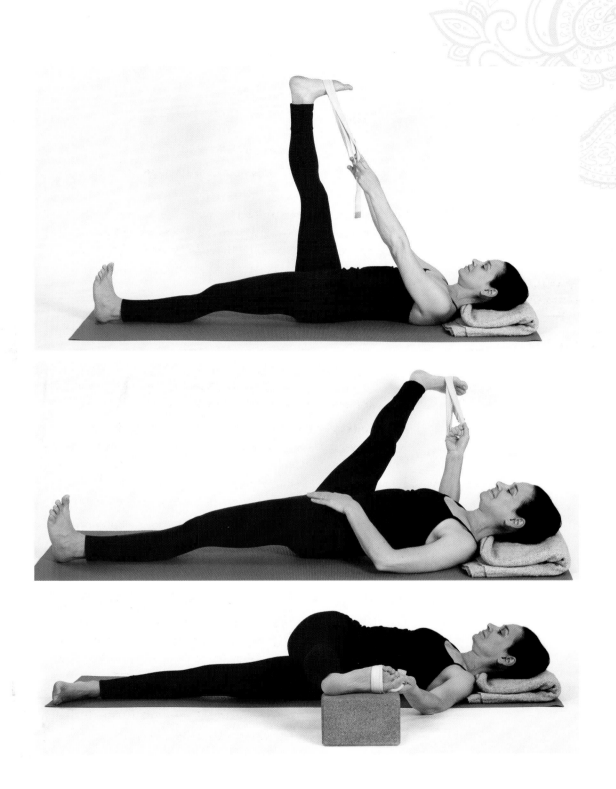

NECK STRETCHES

Chakra Benefited:

Doshic Balance: K–, P+, V+

Your neck holds a lot of tension and stress and this is a great stretch to help to let go of some of that tension. Unlike neck rolls, which are not really very safe for your neck, this stretch is chiropractor approved!

YOU NEED:
- Mat
- Chair (optional)
- 2 blocks (optional)

WHAT TO DO

1. Come to a comfortable seated position either in a chair or on the floor. If needed, put a block under each knee for support.

2. Lengthen your spine and drop your chin to your chest. Roll your right ear toward your right shoulder. Hold for a couple of breaths. You can stretch your left arm away from you to deepen the stretch.

3. Bring your chin back to your chest at center, then roll your left ear toward your left shoulder. Hold for a couple of breaths. Stretch your right arm away from you to deepen the stretch.

4. Bring your chin back to center, and then raise your chin.

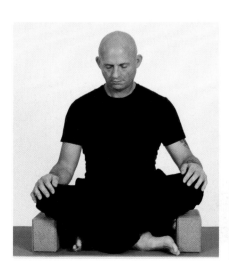
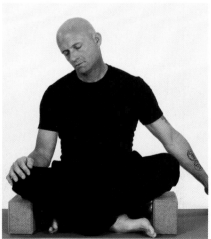
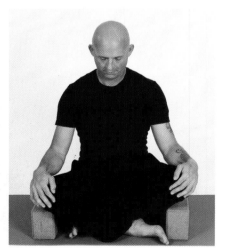

CAT/COW TILTS WITH FEET ON WALL

Chakras Benefited:

Doshic Balance: K–, P+, V+

YOU NEED:

- Mat
- Wall
- Blanket (Head Rest Fold) (optional)

This pose helps you connect with your lower abdominal muscles, which helps to strengthen your lower core, which in turn helps the lower back. Anyone with a tight lower back or lower body issues should use this pose to target this area as they warm up. In addition, this alternative to doing cat/cow on your hands and knees is much easier for people with wrist or knee issues.

WHAT TO DO

1. Lie with your back on the floor and your feet flat on the wall.

2. Bring yourself closer to the wall so that your knees are bent and you look like you are sitting in a chair on your back. Place the blanket under your head for neck support, if needed.

3. Tilt your pelvis so that the back flattens to the floor, and then tilt the other way, creating a curve at the lower back. Continue to do this at least three times. Try to synchronize with breath, exhaling on the cat part (back flat) and inhaling on the cow part (curving back).

YOGIC WISDOM

This pose is a wonderful release for all tension in the back, especially if you spend most of the day sitting at a desk!

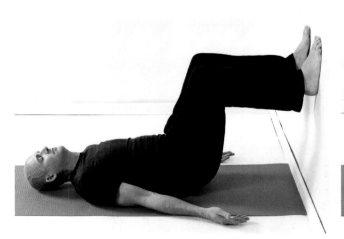
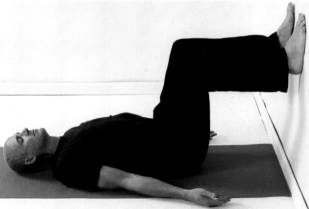

WALL DOWNWARD-FACING DOG

Chakras Benefited:

Doshic Balance: K+, P+, V=

YOU NEED:
- Mat
- Wall or chair

This is a great pose for strengthening the wrists and opening up the shoulders, back, and legs. If you have wrist issues, or you don't like putting too much weight on your hands, doing this pose at the wall helps to relieve the pressure. This is also a wonderful pose for pregnant women, as it allows the uterus to shift, taking pressure off any pinched nerves.

WHAT TO DO

1. Place your hands on the wall or back of a chair and walk backward until your torso is parallel to the floor and your feet are under your hips. Your hands should be shoulder distance apart and in line with your torso.

2. Lean back to make sure that your feet are directly under and in line with your hips, and lower your head between your arms.

3. Hold for at least two minutes to allow enough time for body to release tension.

4. To come out of the pose, walk toward the wall or chair and stand up.

THREADS OF THOUGHT

Viveka-khyātir-aviplavā hānopāyah

Your ability to make distinctions (viveka) between what is changing and what is real; what is fleeting and what is permanent; is the path to the goal of yoga.

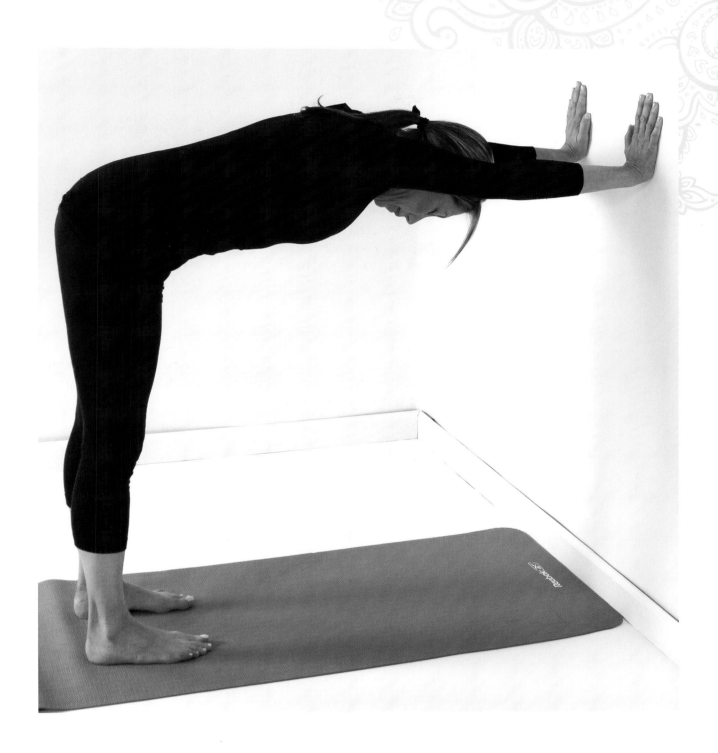

WALL HALF-TRIANGLE FORWARD BEND

Chakras Benefited:

Doshic Balance: K+, P+, V=

YOU NEED:

- Mat
- Wall or chair

This pose loosens and opens the legs and lower back so if you have tight calves or hamstrings, or lower back issues, this is a must for you. The nice part about doing this pose at the wall or chair is that it is safe for almost everyone, even those with blood pressure issues! If you have high blood pressure, you really don't want to invert (meaning let your head go below your heart). It puts undue pressure on the head.

WHAT TO DO

1. Place your hands on the wall or back of a chair. Place your right foot approximately 12 inches from the wall or chair, and step your left foot back about 3 feet, placing it in line with the right foot.

2. Straighten your arms and use the wall or chair for support. Lower your torso parallel halfway toward the floor, keeping your arms in line with your torso. You may need to readjust your stance further back to allow room for your arms to straighten fully. Hold for one minute.

3. Switch your feet, and repeat with the left foot closer to the wall and the right foot 3 feet behind it.

YOGIC WISDOM

As with all forward bends, your back needs to lengthen before you fold from the hips. People often bend from the waist when moving into a forward bend, which is not beneficial, as that is not the area of the back you want the pose to initiate from. You won't get the best stretch, and you could injure yourself. Another thing to note: if you are suffering from lower back pain or have sciatica or disc issues, please keep a bit of a bend in your knees when practicing your forward bend, to protect your back. Remember the no pain = gain concept spoken about in Part 1.

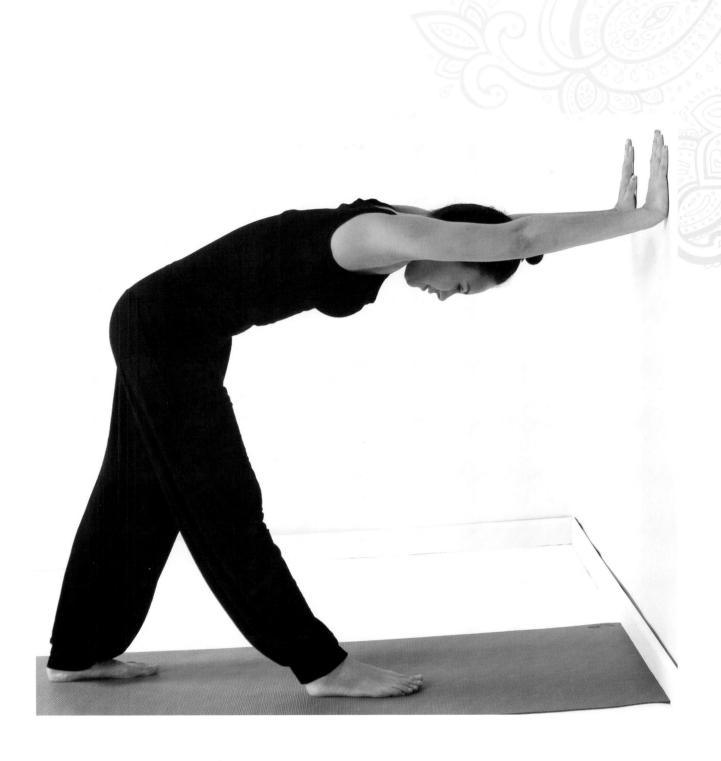

SEATED TWIST

Chakra Benefited:

Doshic Balance: K–, P+, V+

Twists are wonderful for warming up the muscles along the sides of the abdomen (your core) that support your spine and abdominal organs. This particular pose will open up the muscles in your core and lengthen the spine. *Note:* This pose is not recommended if you have spinal stenosis, any bulging spinal disc issues, or if you are pregnant.

FOR OPTION 1 YOU NEED:
- Mat
- Blanket (Small Square or Rectangle Fold) (optional)

OPTION 1

WHAT TO DO

1. Sit in a cross-legged position, with a blanket in the Small Square or Rectangle Fold under your seat for comfort, if desired. Place your left hand on your right knee and bring your right hand behind you. Use your left arm to help you elongate your spine. Inhale as you lengthen and exhale as you deepen the twist. Take at least three full inhales and exhales in this position.

2. Switch the cross of your legs so that the ankle that was along the floor is now on top of the other foot, and repeat on the other side, switching the position of hands and arms as well.

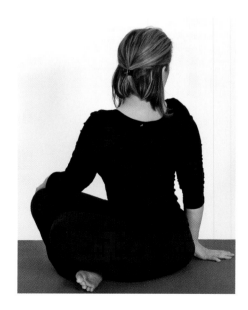

WHAT TO DO

1. Sit on the chair and turn your body so that your legs are facing sideways to the left. If needed, put a block between your knees to protect your back.

2. Bring your hands to the back of the chair, shoulder distance apart. Inhale and lengthen the spine, exhale and twist to the left toward the back of the chair. Do at least three rounds of breaths on this side.

3. Turn your body on the chair so that your legs are facing sideways to the right, and repeat.

FOR OPTION 2 YOU NEED:
- Mat
- Chair
- Block (optional)

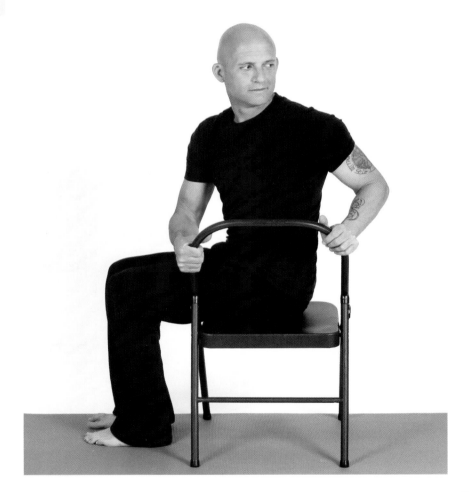

SHOULDER STRETCHES

Chakra Benefited:

Doshic Balance: K–, P+, V+

YOU NEED:
- Mat
- Strap
- Blanket (Small Square or Rectangle Fold) or chair (optional)

Shoulders are complex. The muscles, tendons, bones, sockets, and joints that make up the shoulder can easily become tight or injured with even the simplest movements that you make every day. This series of shoulder stretches helps to warm up and release tension in the shoulder. Whether you overdid it at the gym or you have tension in your neck and shoulders from stress, you can benefit from these stretches. Shoulder stretches even help with headaches! You can do this pose standing, seated on a blanket, or in a chair—whichever is more comfortable.

WHAT TO DO

1. Come to a comfortable seated or standing position. Place your thumbs on the inside of either side of a looped strap the width of your shoulders. Straighten your arms out in front of you.

2. Stretch your arms up overhead as you inhale, and lower them back down in front of you as you exhale. Repeat three times.

3. Straighten your arms out in front of you, then stretch them up overhead. From this position, inhale at center (the midline of your body), exhale and lean to the right, inhale as you move your arms back to the center, then exhale as you lean to the left. Repeat three times on each side, return to the center, then lower your arms.

4. Straighten your arms out in front of you, then stretch them up overhead. From this position, inhale at center (the midline of your body), then exhale and twist to right (try to keep the lower half of the body still). Then inhale as you return to the center, and exhale as you twist to the left. Repeat three times on each side, then return to center and lower your arms.

5. Release one end of the looped strap and bring your hands behind you. Hook your thumbs back into the looped strap, then inhale. Move your arms straight back and up, away from your body as you exhale. Repeat three times.

6. When you complete these stretches, shrug your shoulders up to your ears as you inhale and release them to drop down as you exhale, to release any possible tension that you may still be holding.

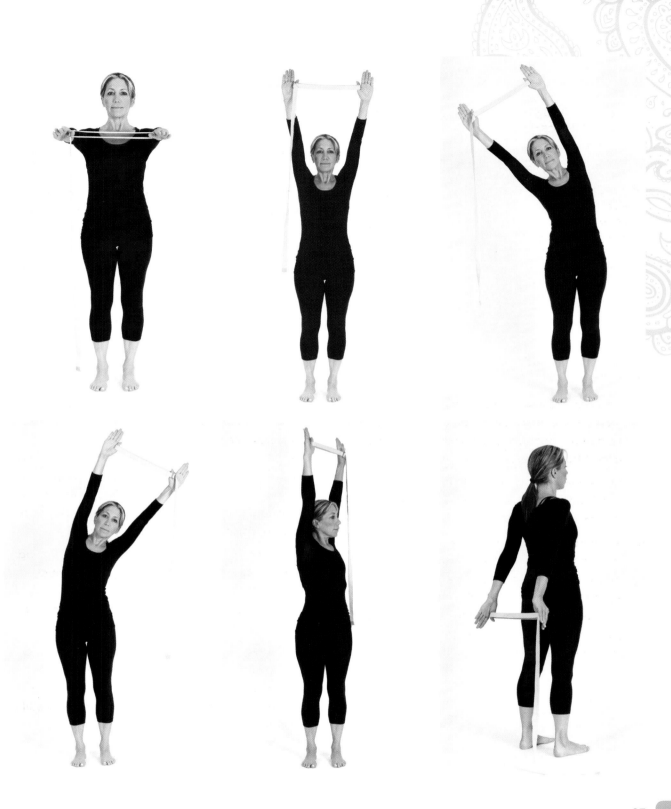

EAGLE ARMS

YOU NEED:
- Mat
- Chair or blanket (Small Square or Rectangle Fold) (optional)

Chakra Benefited:

Doshic Balance: K–, P+, V+

For this pose, you can sit on a blanket (either Small Square or Rectangle Fold) or a chair, or stand. This pose stretches your shoulders and upper back and neck. It's great if you hold tension in these areas, and is a favorite for those who work at a computer all day!

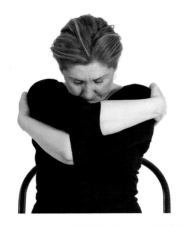

WHAT TO DO

1. Come to a comfortable seated position either in a chair or on the floor, or remain standing. Stretch your arms out to the sides into a T-shape. Cross the right arm across your chest and place it on your left shoulder. Cross your left arm across your chest and place it on your right shoulder.

2. Drop your chin to your chest to stretch the upper back and neck. Breathe there for a couple of breaths, then lift your chin and bend your elbows more, bringing the hands back to back (or palm to palm) by wrapping your arms around each other. Lift the elbows until you feel the stretch and breathe in this position for a couple of breaths. (If your shoulders are very tight, you may not be able to wrap the arms around one another; in this case, it's enough of a stretch to just hold the shoulders where you began.) Release both of your arms to the side and lower them down.

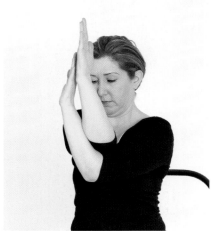

3. Repeat on the other side. Stretch your arms out to the sides in a T-shape, then bring your left hand across to your right shoulder, then your right hand across to the left shoulder. Follow the sequence as written.

COW FACE

YOU NEED:
- Mat
- Chair (optional)
- Blanket (Small Square or Rectangle Fold) or bolster (optional)
- Strap (optional)

Chakra Benefited:

Doshic Balance: K–, P+, V+

This pose stretches the triceps and shoulders. It can helpful to place a blanket or bolster under your buttocks to keep your knees level—it's important to keep your pelvis from tilting forward so that you free up your spine for the stretch.

WHAT TO DO

1. Come to a comfortable seated position either in a chair or on the floor, or remain standing. If sitting, feel free to use a blanket or bolster under your bottom for comfort.

2. Stretch your arms up overhead and bend your right arm, bringing your palm to your upper back as if you were patting yourself on the back. Place your left hand on your right elbow to stretch the tricep muscle. Take a few breaths in this position.

3. Stretch your left arm out to the side and bend your left elbow so that the back of your hand is coming up your back, fingers toward your head. Reach to clasp your right hand. If your hands don't touch, then use a strap or a piece of clothing. Breathe in this position for at least five full breaths in and out.

4. Release your hands and stretch your arms up overhead again, then switch to do the other side.

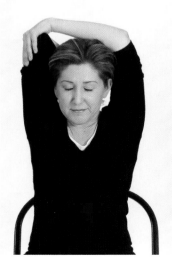
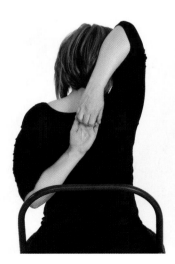
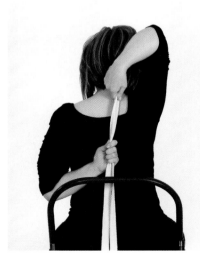

WIND RELIEVING POSE

Chakra Benefited:

Doshic Balance: K+, P+, V=

Wind Relieving Pose is also known as Apanasana because Apana is downward movement, and that is what this pose does; moves energy downward. This pose opens up the digestive tract and relieves tension in the back. Make sure to pay attention to the breath: Inhale as you open up, and exhale as you bring your head toward your knee. Use long, deep breaths.

YOU NEED:
- Mat
- Blanket (Rectangle Fold)

WHAT TO DO

1. Begin by lying on your back on a mat.

2. Inhale, then as you breathe out, hug your right knee in toward you, holding either your shin or your thigh, as you draw your forehead toward your knee. Lower your head as you inhale, and exhale as you lower your leg.

3. Inhale again, and as you breathe out, hug your left knee in toward you, either holding your shin or your thigh, as you draw your forehead toward your knee. Lower your head as you inhale, and lower your leg as you exhale.

4. Repeat three times on each side.

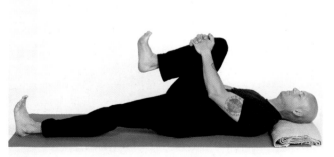

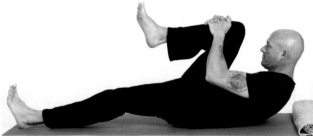

BACK BENDS

In this section you'll find poses that focus on the back and spine—the body's major support system. Back bends help to relieve tension in the back and to counterbalance poor posture, which is a common problem, since many people work at a desk all day. They also stimulate the lymphatic system, which is great for clearing toxins out of the body. One of the most important benefits of back bends in restorative yoga is that they help reduce the flow of cortisol throughout your body, the stress hormone that wreaks so much havoc on our health.

On a physical level, back bends in restorative yoga work and stretch the muscles of the front of the body, but something else very important happens as well—as your front body opens, it allows you to take in a deeper breath, and more energy. As the chest opens, circulation increases to the heart, the nervous system and thymus gland are stimulated, and your metabolism and immune system get a hearty boost. The heart chakra also opens, releasing feelings of fear and grief and replacing them with a greater sense of compassion. What happens during a back bend is that the dullness that you may experience in the mind (in Ayurvedic terms, "tamasic"), which leaves you feeling limited, starts to dissipate and you feel more open to new things, and are able to experience your life more deeply.

For all of these poses, you will lying on the floor, using many props, so be patient! Giving yourself the time to position yourself will help you get the most out of these poses. For any pose, feel free to drape a blanket over your body, use an eye pillow, or use a headwrap to deepen relaxation. The added weight and warmth of these props adds to a sense of security that helps you relax even further.

BLANKET ROLL IN 3 POSITIONS

Chakras Benefited:

Doshic Balance: K–, P+, V+

YOU NEED:
- Mat
- Blanket (Long Roll Fold)

This pose is a great pre-pose for deeper back bends, and is a nice back bend on its own. The posture opens up the back muscles starting at the upper back, moving to the mid-back, and on to the lower back.

WHAT TO DO

1. Lay a mat on the floor.

2. **Position 1:** Place the blanket folded in Long Roll Fold across the middle of your mat. Lie down, positioning yourself so that the blanket roll is below your shoulders (for women, think where the bra strap crosses the back). Your arms should be in a T-shape if possible, and should rest slightly above the rolled blanket, not on the blanket itself. Your knees can be bent or straight, whichever is the most comfortable. Hold this position for two minutes, focusing on your breath and trying to make it as expansive as possible.

3. **Position 2:** Place your hands on the blanket and lift your hips up as you move the blanket down to your mid-back. Carefully lower yourself down onto the roll again. Hold this pose for two minutes. Again, your knees can be bent or straight, whichever is most comfortable. Breathe fully and completely.

4. **Position 3:** Place your hands on the blanket and lift your hips up as you move the blanket to your lower back. Carefully lower yourself down onto the roll and relax there for two minutes.

5. When the two minutes are up, lift your hips and remove the blanket, then lower your back to the mat again, keeping your knees bent. As you prepare to transition to sit up, let your knees knock into each other with your feet more widely spread, and let your back relax for a minute before you get up. Roll to your right side and come up to a sitting position.

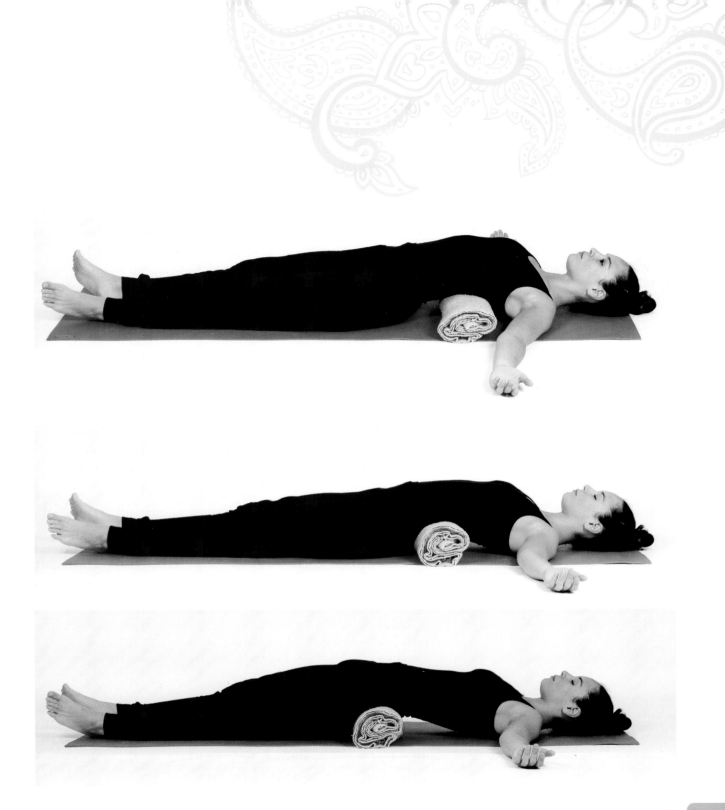

SIMPLE BRIDGE WITH BLOCK OR BOLSTER UNDER HIPS

Chakra Benefited:

Doshic Balance: K–, P+, V+

YOU NEED:
- Mat
- Block or bolster

This pose is for when you've been sitting all day. It counters all the tension that accumulates in the lower back. It's a nice release, especially if you suffer from sacroiliac joint dysfunction, or just have a lot of lower back tension in general.

WHAT TO DO

1. Lie down on the mat. Bend your knees, lift your hips, and place either a block (at any height that feels right) or a bolster under your lower back.

2. Lower yourself onto the support of your choice. Relax with your arms resting on the floor next to your body with the palms facing up.

3. Breathe and relax. Stay here for a minimum of three minutes to a maximum of eight minutes.

4. To come out of this pose, lift your hips and remove the prop. Lower yourself to the floor and rest there for a few moments. Roll to your right side to come up.

VARIATION

If you don't have a block or a bolster, you can use a few blankets instead. Fold them using the Rectangle Fold and stack them, depending on how high you want to go.

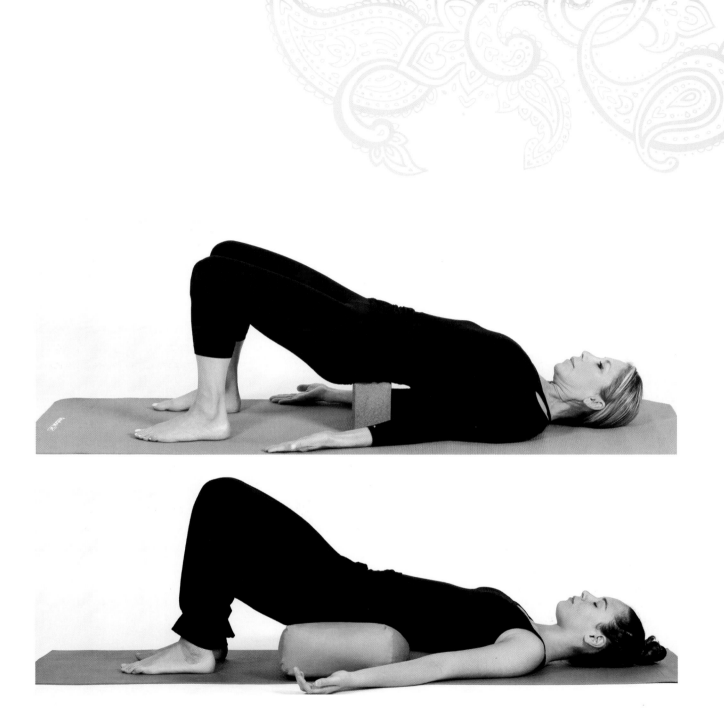

RECLINING BRIDGE POSE

Chakra Benefited:

Doshic Balance: K−, P+, V+

This pose is great for opening the upper back, dispelling lung congestion, and opening the heart chakra. If you experience pain in your lower back, explore this pose with knees bent and feet on the floor.

FOR OPTION 1 YOU NEED:
- Mat
- 2 bolsters the same size (the less open you are, the better off you are using a rectangular bolster, since it's lower) (if you don't have bolsters, you can use blankets in their place [Rectangle Fold])
- Blanket (Head Rest or Rectangle Fold) (optional)
- 2 blankets (Small Square Fold) (optional)
- Strap (optional)

FOR OPTION 2 YOU NEED:
- Wall
- Mat
- 2 blocks
- Bolster
- Blanket (Head Rest or Rectangle Fold) (optional)

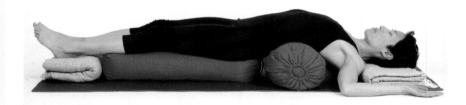

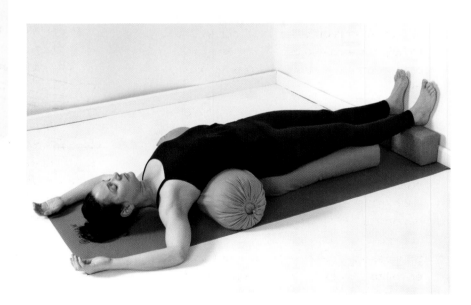

WHAT TO DO

1. Place the bolsters or blankets in the Rectangle Fold on the mat. Align them in the shape of a long rectangle, roughly paralleling where your body will be, from the mid-back to the feet. Alternatively, you may arrange them in a T-shape, depending on how it feels when you lie down. Lie down so that your shoulder blades come over the end of the bolster and your head rests on the floor (or on a blanket in the Head Rest or Rectangle Fold). The second bolster (or folded blanket in the Small Square Fold) should support your knees and calves. Arms should extend out from the body in a T-shape, or gently curved slightly away from the body to create a U-shape.

2. It's possible your legs will be long enough to need a small blanket in the Small Square Fold to support your feet. You may also choose to strap your legs onto the bolster on your thighs to help the legs and back relax. Bring the strap around your legs and the bolster to provide the most support.

3. To come out of this pose, place your feet on the floor and lift your hips, pushing the bolster away from you with your hands until your buttocks can rest on the floor. Place your feet on the bolster; let your feet come together as your knees drop out to each side. This is a nice hip opener, and a way to relax the back before you move on. Hold this position for one minute, then use your hands to bring your legs together, roll to your right side, and press up into a sitting position.

WHAT TO DO

1. Face the wall on the mat. Place two blocks at medium height up against the wall. Then place a bolster underneath you, the narrow end toward the wall, and sit on it. You will have to adjust the distance between the end of the bolster and the wall to accommodate your height. Place your feet up against the wall with your heels resting on the blocks, then lie down on the bolster. Push yourself back until your shoulders are over the other end of the bolster and your head is resting on the floor (or the optional folded blanket, if desired). Legs should be fully outstretched, the feet pressing firmly into the wall. Your arms should rest on the floor in a T- or U-shape. Hold this pose for a minimum of five minutes and for as long as twenty minutes.

2. To come out of this pose, bend your knees and place your feet on the floor. Lifting your hips, push the bolster away from you and toward the wall until your buttocks can come to rest on the floor. Place your feet on the bolster, then let your feet come together and your knees drop out to each side. This opens the hips and relaxes the back before you move on. Hold this pose for one minute, then use your hands to lift your knees and bring your legs together. Roll to your right side, and press up into a sitting position.

SUPPORTED BOUND ANGLE POSE

Chakras Benefited:

Doshic Balance: K–, P–, V=

FOR OPTION 1 YOU NEED:
- Mat
- Bolster
- Blanket (Head Rest Fold) (optional)
- 2 blankets (Short Roll Fold) (optional)

FOR OPTION 2 YOU NEED:
- Mat
- 2 blocks
- Bolster
- Blanket (Head Rest Fold) (optional)
- 2 blankets (Short Roll Fold) (optional)
- Blanket (Open Fold) (optional)

This pose is a favorite in restorative yoga. It creates a sense of calm as it opens up the back and the hips, stretches your inner thighs, and opens up your pelvic area. It is a very prop-heavy pose, so refer to Chapter 3 to learn how to set up the props for each option. For added relaxation, drape a blanket over you.

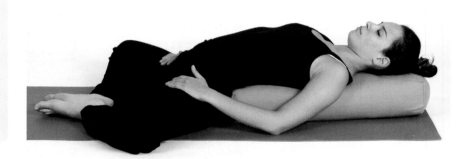

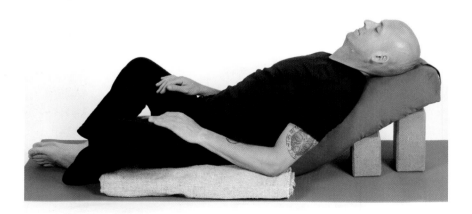

WHAT TO DO

1. Place a bolster lengthwise on your mat.

2. Sit on the floor and bring your lower back right up to the narrow end of the bolster.

3. Place your hands on the bolster behind you, pull your chest forward in a slight back bend, and lie back over the bolster.

4. Bring the soles of your feet together and let your knees drop out to the sides.

5. If you need more support under your neck, use the blanket in the Head Rest Fold and place under your head. If you need more support for your legs, take two blankets in the Short Roll Fold and use them as mini bolsters under your knees. You can rest your hands on your thighs or let your arms rest alongside you, with your palms facing up. Stay in this pose for a minimum of five minutes to a maximum of a half hour.

6. To come out of this pose, bring your legs together with your hands by pressing against the outside of your thighs. Roll to your right side and come up to sit after adjusting for a few moments.

WHAT TO DO

1. On your mat, place a pair of two blocks a short distance apart. The pair can consist of either a tall and a medium height block, or a medium and a short height block. Place a bolster on the blocks.

2. Sit on the floor and bring your lower back right up to the lower narrow end of the bolster.

3. Place your hands on the bolster behind you, pull your chest forward in a slight back bend, and lie back over the bolster.

4. Bring the soles of your feet together and let your knees drop out to the sides.

5. If you need more support under your neck, place the blanket in the Head Rest Fold under your head. If you need more support for your legs, take two blankets in the Short Roll Fold and use them as mini bolsters under your knees. You may also use the Open Fold blanket to drape over your whole body. Rest your hands on your thighs or let your arms rest next to you with your palms facing up.

6. To come out of this pose, bring your legs together by pressing your hands against the outside of your thighs. Roll to your right side and come up to sit after adjusting for a few moments.

WHAT TO DO

1. Set the bolster up either flat (as in Option 1) or at an angle (as in Option 2).

2. Bring your lower back right up to the narrow end of the bolster. Place your hands on the bolster behind you, pull your chest forward in a slight back bend, and lie back over the bolster.

3. Take a strap and fasten it into a wide loop. Bring the loop over your head and position it around your back, right below your waist. Bring the soles of your feet together and let your knees drop out to the sides.

4. Place your feet facing each other inside the other end of the strap loop, and lift the side of the loop so that they rest over the inside of your thighs. Tighten the looped strap until your bent knees feel supported. Rest your hands on your thighs or let your arms rest next to you with your palms facing up.

5. If you need more support under your neck, use the blanket in the Head Rest Fold under your head. If you need more support for your legs, take two blankets in the Short Roll Fold and use them as mini bolsters under your knees.

6. To come out of this pose, bring your legs together by pressing your hands against the outside of your thighs. Roll to your right side and come up to sit after adjusting for a few moments.

FOR OPTION 3 YOU NEED:

- Mat
- Bolster
- 2 blocks (optional)
- Strap
- Blanket (Head Rest Fold) (optional)
- 2 blankets (Short Roll Fold) (optional)

VARIATION

In Option 3, instead of placing strap around your back as in Step 3, place looped strap around your bent knees, bring soles of feet together, and let knees drop out to the side, supported by the strap.

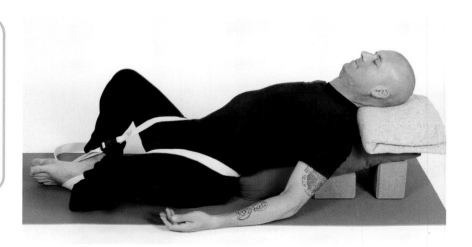

WHAT TO DO

1. Set the bolster up either flat (as in Option 1) or at an angle (as in Option 2). Place your hands on the bolster behind you, pull your chest forward in a slight back bend, and lie back over the bolster.

2. Take another bolster and place it perpendicular to the first bolster, under your knees.

3. Bring the soles of your feet together and let your knees drop out to the sides, supported by the bolster. Rest your hands on your thighs or let your arms rest next to you with your palms facing up.

4. If you need more support under your neck, use the blanket in the Head Rest Fold under your head.

5. If you choose to explore the swaddled option with a blanket over you, with your arms straight out in front of you, drape the blanket in the Open Fold lengthwise across your arms. Then fold the blanket under your arms so that when you lower your arms they are encompassed by the blanket for support.

6. To come out of this pose, bring your legs together by pressing your hands against the outside of your thighs. Roll to your right side and come up to sit after adjusting for a few moments.

FOR OPTION 4 YOU NEED:
- Mat
- 2 bolsters
- 2 blocks (optional)
- Blanket (Head Rest Fold) (optional)
- Blanket (Open Fold) (optional, for swaddling)

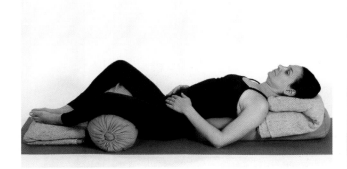

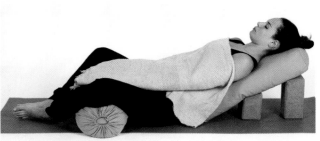

FOR OPTION 5 YOU NEED:

- Mat
- Bolster
- 2 blocks (optional)
- Blanket (Oblong Fold)
- Blanket (Head Rest Fold) (optional)

YOGIC WISDOM

The Supported Bound Angle Pose is great for women when they are experiencing PMS and menopause symptoms, as it helps to release tension. It is also beneficial for those who have digestion problems, as it stimulates the abdominal organs and aids digestion. It opens up tight hips, and is also a beneficial pose for the back.

WHAT TO DO

1. Set the bolster up either flat (as in Option 1) or at an angle on blocks (as in Option 2), and keep a blanket in the Oblong Fold at your side.

2. Place your hands on the bolster behind you, pull your chest forward in a slight back bend, and lie back over the bolster. If you need more support under your neck, place the Head Rest Fold blanket under your head.

3. Bring the soles of your feet together and place a blanket in the Oblong Fold horizontally so it wraps around the top of your feet. Thread the ends of the folded blanket out and down around your legs, and then up through your legs. Pull the ends of the blanket toward you so that your feet come closer to your groin, and let your knees drop out to the sides. Allow the ends of the folded blanket to rest over your thighs.

4. To come out of this pose, bring your legs together by pressing your hands against the outside of your thighs. Slide your feet out of the blanket, roll to your right side, and come up to sit after adjusting for a few moments.

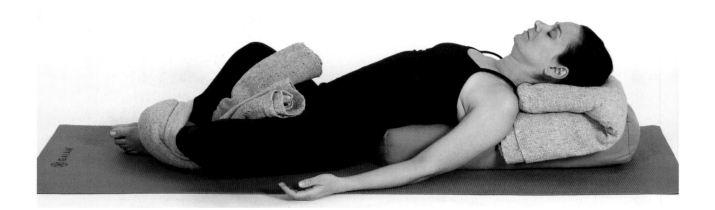

CROSS BOLSTER POSE

Chakras Benefited:

Doshic Balance: K−, P+, V+

This pose is an easy back bend: easy to set up, and easy on the body physically. It can soothe your heart when you're not feeling in the best spirits, as it opens the front of the body and the heart chakra. Doing this pose with your feet pressed into the wall can add a sense of comfort and stability.

YOU NEED:

- Mat
- 2 bolsters (preferably a round and a flat, using the round on the bottom)
- Blanket (Head Rest Fold) (optional)

VARIATION

If you only have one bolster, then use one or two blankets (Rectangle Fold) in place of the bolster on the bottom.

WHAT TO DO

1. On your mat, cross the bolsters at their middle to make a plus sign shape. Lie on them with the bolster on top parallel to your spine and the bottom bolster parallel to your outstretched arms. Your hips should be the highest point of your body. Drape your shoulders over the top end of the vertical bolster. Keep your arms in a U-shape, or spread out in a T-shape. Rest your head on the floor, or support it with a blanket in a Head Rest Fold, if needed. Hold the pose for at least five minutes.

2. To come out of the pose, slide yourself toward your feet until your bottom is off the bolster and on the floor. Bend your knees and then roll to your right, and slowly come up to sit.

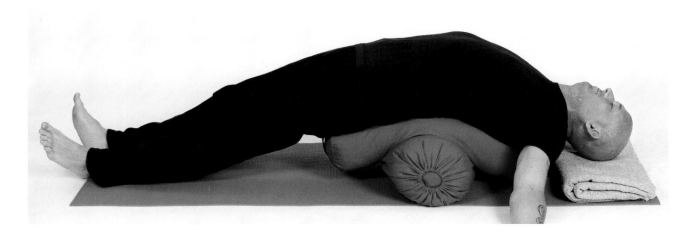

FISH POSE
WITH BLOCKS OR BOLSTER

Chakra Benefited:

Doshic Balance: K–, P+, V+

YOU NEED:
- Mat
- 2 blocks
- 1–2 bolsters (optional)
- Headwrap (optional)

The thymus gland (located in the chest behind the upper breastbone) is the center of the immune system, so if the thymus gland is stimulated, then so is the immune system. Poses that open the chest, such as Fish Pose, help to build your immune system so it can attack invaders, such as viruses and bacteria, with more strength. But Fish Pose, when done in restorative yoga, can also calm the immune system, which particularly helps when the immune system is in overdrive during allergy season. If you practice this pose with only one block under your back, this pose opens the throat as well. Breathe deeply into the chest during Fish Pose to get the most benefit. This pose can be done with the blocks alone, or with a bolster laid over them.

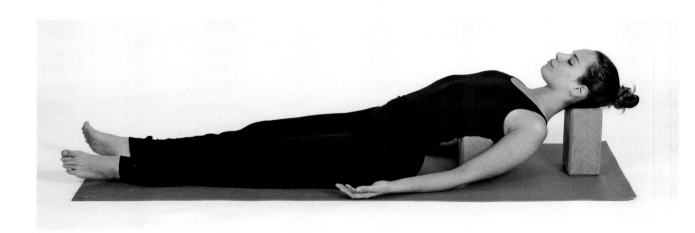

WHAT TO DO

1. If you are using blocks, place two blocks a short distance apart on your mat. The pair can consist of either a tall and a medium height block, or a medium and a short height block. If you're using a bolster, either lay one bolster over the blocks, or lay the bolster flat on the mat.

2. Lie back over the blocks or bolster, legs outstretched in front of you. Stay for at least five minutes, and focus on your breath and opening your chest. Feel free to use a headwrap for comfort and additional relaxation, if desired. If you wish, you may bend your legs and place a second bolster underneath them for support. Rest your arms alongside your body with your palms facing up or toward your body.

3. To come out, bend your knees and roll to your side. Push the blocks and/or bolsters out of the way and roll back onto your back, keeping your knees bent. Feel the more open sensation you have created in your chest area. When you have adjusted, roll to your side and come up to sit.

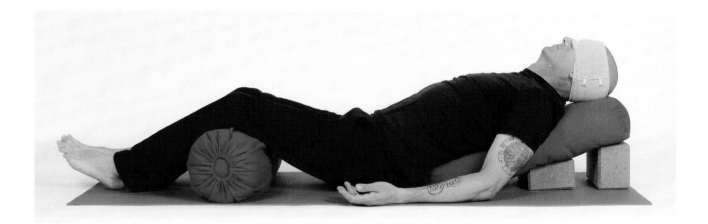

HEART OPENING POSE

Chakra Benefited:

Doshic Balance: K–, P–, V=

YOU NEED:
- Mat
- 2 bolsters
- Blanket (Head Rest Fold or Rectangle Fold) (optional)

This pose helps to counteract all of the hunching forward that you likely do every day (think of all the times in one day: at your desk, in the car, and more!). This pose opens up the back and chest, and helps to free your breath to bring fresh energy throughout your body. Overall, it's a very invigorating pose, especially as you come out of it. Note that this particular pose uses double horizontal bolsters. Some of the sequences that use this pose only require one bolster or a blanket. See the specific instructions in the sequences to know which props to use and when.

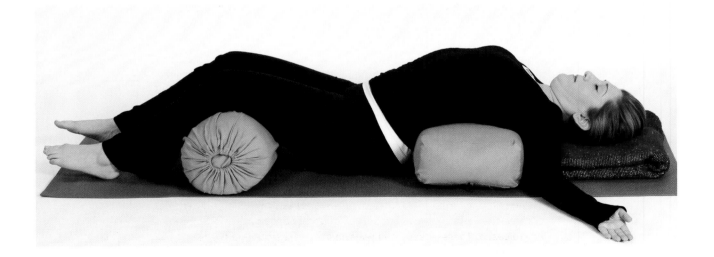

WHAT TO DO

1. Place one bolster across the mat to go under your shoulder blades and mid-back area, and another bolster across the mat to go under your knees.

2. Lie over the bolsters with your arms out in a T-shape above the top of the bolster under your shoulders. If the bolster feels too high, you can place a Head Rest Fold blanket under your head, or swap the first bolster for a Rectangle Fold blanket under your shoulders.

3. Hold this position for a minimum of five minutes and a maximum of twenty minutes. Focus on breathing fully and deeply into your chest.

4. To come out of the pose, place your feet on the bolster that is positioned under your knees, and push the bolster away. With knees bent, roll to your right side. At this point, you can push the upper bolster toward your head and use it as a pillow, if you like. Allow yourself a few moments to adjust, and then come up to sit.

YOGIC WISDOM

Have you ever caught yourself sitting with your chest collapsed, shoulders rounded? It's a sure sign that something is off—you may be feeling depressed, unenthusiastic, or tired. When your heart chakra (Anahata) is closed, your chest collapses, your breathing may be shallow, and energy simply isn't being allowed to flow through your heart and lungs as openly and freely as it does in your natural state. When performing back bend poses in restorative yoga, your chest is allowed to open, energy begins to flow, and deep tensions in this area are released. These poses open your heart, and restore you to the loving, exuberant human being you are.

RECLINING HERO POSE

Chakras Benefited:

Doshic Balance: K+, P+, V=

FOR OPTION 1 YOU NEED:

- Mat
- Bolster
- Blanket (Square Fold) (optional)
- Blanket (Rectangle Fold) (optional)
- Block (optional)

FOR OPTION 2 YOU NEED:

- Mat
- 2–4 blocks (2 mandatory, 2 optional)
- Bolster
- 2 blankets (Long Roll Fold)

Tight back? You may be surprised to learn that tight quadriceps may be the culprit! Reclining Hero Pose stretches the quadriceps, abdomen, and the deep hip flexor, which can be a real antidote to lower back tension. Not only is this pose beneficial for back issues, it also helps with your breathing and digestion. If you have tight quadriceps muscles or knee issues, it will be challenging, but with the props used in restorative yoga, it becomes easier! This posture can be modified, depending on your needs. For each variation, stay in the position for at least five minutes.

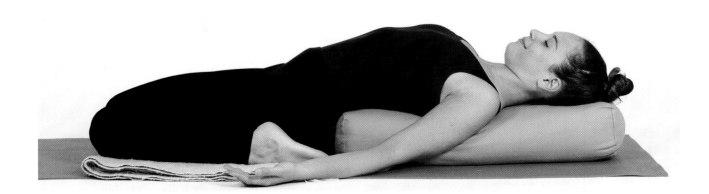

WHAT TO DO

1. If desired, place a blanket in the Square Fold on the mat for extra padding. Kneel and open your knees slightly. With the bolster flat on the mat and parallel to your spine behind you, place your hands on it and lie back onto it. You may need to raise your head slightly; place a blanket (Rectangle Fold) under your head if needed. If this is even slightly uncomfortable, raise the end of the bolster that is under your head with one block, so the bolster is on an angle. Your arms should rest alongside you, with the palms facing up.

2. Come out of this pose onto your hands and knees by pressing your hands into the floor and pushing up to sit upright. Then stretch one leg backward at a time to restore circulation to your legs.

WHAT TO DO

1. If Option 1 is too much of a stretch, kneel and rest your buttocks on a block at the short or medium height in front of the bolster, and place another block (at whichever height feels comfortable) under the head end of the bolster to angle it before you lie back on the bolster. If you need the bolster raised more, place a block at the short or medium height under the end at the base of your spine and a block at medium or tall height under the head end to maintain the angle. Place one blanket in the Long Roll Fold along each of your sides to act as arm-rests.

2. Come out of this pose onto your hands and knees by pressing your hands into the floor and pushing up to sit upright. Then stretch one leg backward at a time to restore circulation to your legs.

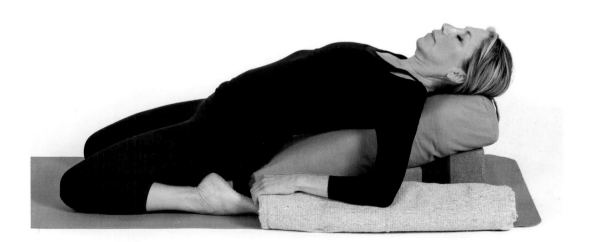

WHAT TO DO

FOR OPTION 3 YOU NEED:
- Mat
- Chair
- Wall
- 2 bolsters (one may only be necessary, it depends on the length of your torso)
- 4 blocks (you may not need them all, but it's helpful to have handy if you find you need extra support)
- 2 blankets (Rectangle Fold)
- Blanket (Square Fold)
- Blanket (Small Square Fold) (optional)

1. Place the back of a chair against the wall, on the mat. Place a blanket in a Square Fold on your mat, in front of your chair. Prop your bolster(s) on an angle with the top narrow end where your head will go, leaning on the seat of the chair. Place a block at medium height under the middle of the bolster to help support it. Place another block at short height on the mat in front of where the bolster touches the floor. Kneel with your knees apart slightly, and lower your buttocks to rest on this short block. Place two blocks at short or medium height next to you, one on each side, and place a blanket in a Rectangle Fold on each block. Lie back onto the bolster and rest your arms on the blanket-covered blocks, placing your hands on your abdomen, or resting them at your sides. It's possible you will need additional props, depending on the length of your torso. If that is the case, place a bolster on the seat of the chair horizontally, and if you need additional support a blanket in a Small Square Fold to support your head as well.

2. Come out of this pose onto your hands and knees by pressing your hands into the floor and pushing up to sit upright. Then stretch one leg backward at a time to restore circulation to your legs.

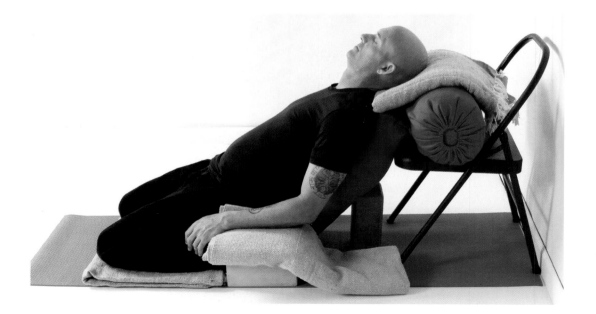

TWISTS

Twists are some of the most valuable yoga poses for your body. From a physical standpoint, twists keep the spine and major joints (including those in the hips and shoulders) in good working order. Too often, people lose mobility in their spine due to living in a sedentary culture. The tissue along the spinal column and in the joints shortens from underuse, it becomes more painful to do ordinary motions, and your body becomes more susceptible to injury. It's a losing situation that practicing twist poses can slow down.

Along with benefiting the spine, twists help to squeeze and tone the abdominal organs, and help maintain the nervous and circulatory systems as well. Iyengar describes twists as having a "squeeze-and-soak" effect on the organs. Think of your body as a washcloth from which you are wringing out excess water: as you squeeze your inner organs during a twist, toxin-rich blood is squeezed out of the organs and new fresh blood is allowed to flow in. Twists stimulate the fresh flow of circulation and encourage the nervous system to refresh itself—plus, they just feel good!

Using one of these poses each day is a good way to keep your body supple and flexible. Twists are especially good as transitional poses between forward and back bends as they warm up the spine and stimulate fresh blood flow to the muscles and organs.

YOGIC WISDOM

Most restorative twists are safe for everyone, but it is important to consider a few things. If you recently have had abdominal surgery, it is important to check with your doctor first before doing these poses. If you have sciatica or sacroiliac joint pain, practice these poses with as many modifications (extra blankets and blocks) as needed for support so that you do not feel any pain. For pregnant women, twists are not usually advised in active yoga classes, but in restorative yoga, they are safe. Use props to help you remain comfortable and supported.

REVOLVED ABDOMEN POSE

Chakras Benefited:

Doshic Balance: K−, P+, V+

Revolved Abdomen Pose can be one of the most satisfying poses in yoga. The pressure of the body against itself as you twist allows a natural release without much effort. The lower back and abdominal muscles get a healthy squeeze in this pose, and give the digestive organs a healthy boost. In restorative yoga, this twist is done with your hips raised on a bolster for added support. While you are in the pose, be receptive to releasing all the toxins in your core. (If the bolster is too high for your hips in this pose, substitute a Rectangle Fold blanket instead.)

WHAT TO DO

1. Place a bolster across your mat, about halfway down. Sit in the middle of the bolster, then turn and lie down on your left side with your bottom arm parallel to the bolster by bringing your legs up toward your chest with your knees bent. Let your right leg fully cross over your body so that your left knee comes to rest toward the floor. Your right hip will be in the air, while your left will be on the bolster. Place a second bolster between your legs. Add a Rectangle Fold blanket under your bottom leg, if you need the additional support. You are working to twist your torso and legs to a 90-degree angle across the floor, so remember to twist from your torso, not your knees.

YOU NEED:
- Mat
- 2 bolsters
- Blanket (Rectangle Fold) (optional)
- Blanket (Head Rest Fold) (optional)

YOGIC WISDOM

Keep plenty of props nearby (blankets of different folds, blocks) and use them generously to get the full benefits of the pose. Make sure that your head, pelvis, knees, and feet feel fully supported.

2. Open your arms in a T-shape and lie back so that your back, head, and arms rest on the floor. Be sure to keep your hips and legs in the initial position. If your head is uncomfortable, support it by placing a blanket in the Head Rest Fold under it. If your right shoulder is uncomfortable, keep your right hand on your ribs, relaxing your elbow toward the ground. Hold this position for at least three minutes.

3. To come out of pose, bring your right arm over to the left side and push up to sit, letting your head come up last. Repeat the pose on the other side.

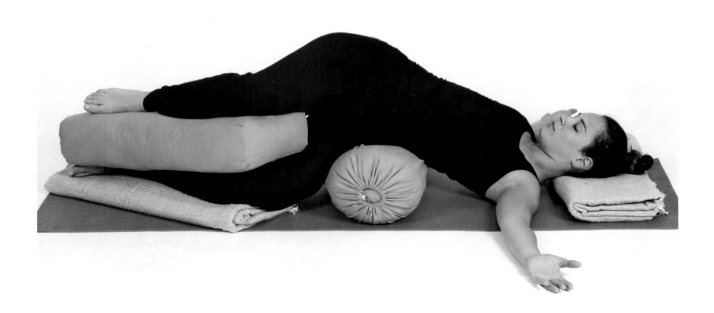

BELLY DOWN TWIST OVER BOLSTER

Chakra Benefited:

Doshic Balance: K–, P+, V+

This pose is a relaxing twist where you can feel fully at rest. It relieves stress and tension in the muscles along the sides and midsection of the torso, which relaxes your breathing as well, contributing to an overall feeling of peace. This gentle pose is really for everyone, even those with back problems or those who are pregnant, so don't let yourself be intimidated.

YOU NEED:
- Mat
- Bolster
- 2 blocks (optional)
- 2–4 blankets (Rectangle Fold) (optional)

WHAT TO DO

1. Place the bolster lengthwise along the middle of your mat. Keep your blankets and blocks nearby.

2. Sit in front of the bolster, then bring your right hip up to the bolster with your knees bent, and allow them to fall in a comfortable position.

3. Experiment with the bolster to make sure you feel comfortable and supported. You may choose to raise the bolster on an angle by using blocks (use a short and medium pair, or medium and tall pair), and/or place a Rectangle Fold blanket across the bolster underneath your head for support.

4. Stretch your bottom arm along the bolster and then lower your arm to the floor next to it. Place your top hand on the other side of the bolster. Turn your belly toward the bolster and lower yourself down to the bolster. As you do inhale and lengthen your spine, then exhale and twist a little more. Turn your head either toward your knees, or, for a deeper twist, away from your knees. If you did not turn away from your knees initially, you may find

YOGIC WISDOM

Though the pose is a "closed twist" (meaning you are closing the spaces within your body) and usually contraindicated for pregnancy, it is actually an accepted twist if you are pregnant. If you are pregnant, just leave space between your hip and the bolster for your belly.

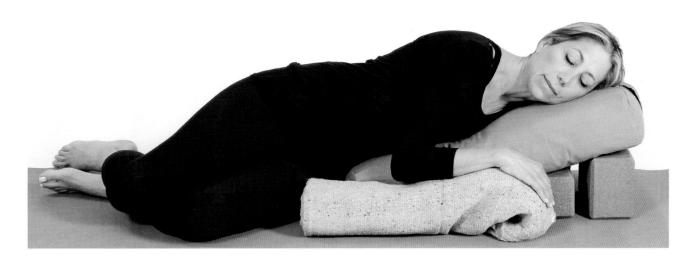

that after a few minutes you can turn your head to the deeper twist side as your body relaxes. Let the bolster support you: Relax your arms and try not to hold yourself up. If you need to, place a blanket or block between your knees to take any strain off the back if you feel it. You may also prop up your arms on two Rectangle Fold blankets at a slight angle, so that your hands are higher than your elbows for even more comfort.

5. Hold this position for three minutes, then come out of the pose by pressing yourself away from the bolster with your hands on the floor and sitting up. Repeat on the left side.

SCISSORED LEGS BELLY DOWN TWIST

Chakra Benefited:

Doshic Balance: K–, P+, V+

YOU NEED:
- Mat
- Bolster
- 2 blocks (optional)
- 2–4 blankets (Rectangle Fold) (optional)

Closed twists such as this tend to provide a deeper pressure on the abdominal organs than open twists, since they compress the spaces within the body. This pose provides a little bit more of a stretch on the side of your lower leg, and while restorative poses should be relaxing, sometimes a little extra stretch can ultimately help your body relax more deeply. Everyone can do this pose to some degree, but it is especially good for runners and cyclers, as it helps to open up the iliotibial band, the ligament that often becomes aggravated during running and cycling.

WHAT TO DO

1. Place the bolster lengthwise along the middle of your mat. Keep your blankets and blocks nearby.

2. Sit in front of the bolster, then bring your right hip up to the bolster with your knees bent.

3. Extend your lower leg out so it is perpendicular to the bolster. Straighten your top leg so that it is in line with your torso.

4. Place your hands to each side of the bolster, and turn your belly toward the bolster. Lower yourself down to the bolster, turning your head either toward your top leg, or, for a deeper twist, away from your top leg. If you did not turn away initially, you may find that after a few minutes you can turn your head to the deeper twist side as your body relaxes.

THREADS OF THOUGHT

Abhyāsa-vairāgya-ābhyāṁ tan-nirodha

To experience a state of yoga, you both need dedicated action (abhyasa) and detachment or surrender (vairagya). Like the two wings of a bird, you need both to fly.

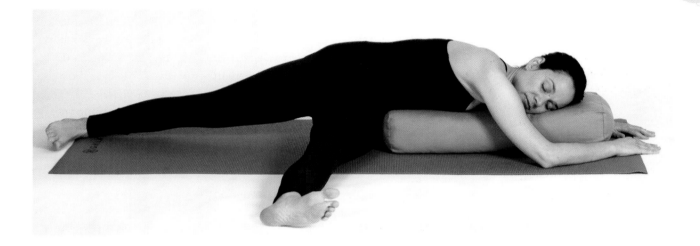

5. Experiment with the bolster to make sure your back feels aligned and comfortable as it rests on it. You may choose to raise the bolster on an angle by using blocks (use a short and medium pair, or medium and large pair), and/or place a Rectangle Fold blanket widthwise across the mat underneath your head for support.

6. Let yourself be supported by the bolster; relax your arms and try not to hold yourself up. You may choose to bend your legs slightly to remove any strain that doesn't feel comfortable. Hold this pose for at least three minutes.

7. To come out of the pose, press yourself away from the bolster with your hands pressing into the floor and sit up. Repeat on the left side.

SIDE LYING STRETCH

Chakras Benefited:

Doshic Balance: K–, P+, V+

Although this pose is not technically a twist, it does open the side body, which makes it a nice, easy transition into a twist pose. This Side Lying Stretch helps with stagnant energy in the body. If someone is feeling as if his or her energy is low, this is a great pose to get the energy moving again. Also, if you are dealing with gallbladder issues, this is a wonderful pose to spend time in regularly.

YOU NEED:

- Mat
- Bolster or blanket (Short Roll Fold)
- Blanket (Rectangle Fold) (optional)

WHAT TO DO

1. Place a bolster or Short Roll Fold blanket across the middle of your mat and sit down with your left hip against it, facing the long side of your mat.

2. Stretch your left leg out so it lies along the floor perpendicular to the bolster. Straighten your right leg so it is in line with your torso and lower leg.

3. Stretch your left arm up straight above your head. Lie down on your left side with the bolster under the side of your upper chest, and rest your head on your arm (you may need a Rectangle Fold blanket under your arm to raise it up a bit). Reach your right arm up over your head so that it is in line with your left arm. Your arms will be parallel to the floor, flanking your ears.

4. Let yourself be supported by the bolster or blanket; relax your arms and try not to hold yourself up. You may choose to bend your legs slightly to remove any strain that doesn't feel comfortable. Hold this position for three minutes.

5. To come out of the pose, place your hands on the floor, press yourself away from the bolster, and sit up. Repeat on the other side.

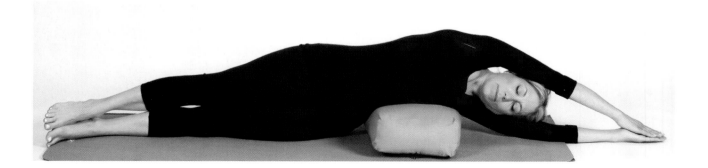

FORWARD BENDS

Forward bends are poses of surrender, and are therefore very calming. They create this feeling by curling the body forward and opening up the back area of the body, forming a "shell" shape where you feel supported in yourself. Because most forward bends gently massage the belly, they improve digestion and, if needed, can help with women's issues such as menstrual cramps and infertility. Forward bends are also good for relieving insomnia, and have been known to help lower high blood pressure. Many forward bends position the head below the heart or parallel to the heart, which symbolizes letting go of the ego and allowing your heart to guide your decisions, which encourages an even a deeper connection to your soul.

CHILD'S POSE

Chakras Benefited:

Doshic Balance: K+, P+, V–

For OPTION 1 YOU NEED:
- Mat
- Blanket (Half Fold) (optional)
- Blanket (Square Fold)
- 1–2 bolsters (a second bolster is sometimes necessary for more support)
- 2 blocks (optional)
- Blanket (Long Roll Fold) (optional)
- 2 blankets (Rectangle Fold) (optional)

FOR OPTION 2 YOU NEED:
- Mat
- 2 chairs
- 1–2 bolsters
- 1–2 blocks

Child's Pose is the cornerstone rest pose in yoga. It's a "safe" pose, where you will come to feel supported and nurtured and able to connect with your breath. On a physical level, Child's Pose is a great forward bend that helps to gently open up the back of the body while also giving the abdominal organs a massage. It's important that you don't feel like you are holding yourself up in this posture—let the bolster or chairs do the work of supporting you so that you can fully relax.

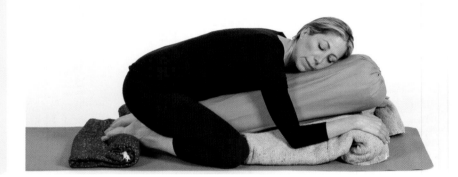

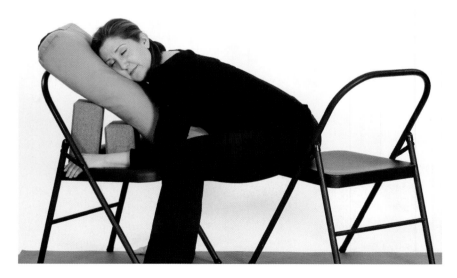

WHAT TO DO

1. If you need extra padding under your knees, place a blanket with a Half Fold (folded lengthwise) on the floor. If you have tight feet, keep a Square Fold blanket nearby for under the tops of your feet. You can roll the blanket up as much as you need for comfort.

2. Place the narrow end of the bolster between your knees and sit back to rest on your heels. Fold forward and rest your whole belly on the bolster. You may raise the bolster higher by using two blocks at either short and medium height or medium and tall height to angle the bolster by placing the blocks so they support the middle and head of the bolster. If desired, place a Long Roll Fold blanket at the crease of your hip and thigh to create additional support for the low back.

3. If your arms do not rest comfortably on the floor, or they don't reach the floor, place a Rectangle Fold blanket under each arm. You can turn the top of the blanket under to make a nice resting spot for your hands.

4. Turn your head to one side, and then after a few minutes turn your head to the other side. Spend the same amount of time on each side.

5. Stay in the posture for at least five minutes. When you are finished, gently uncurl your body, move the bolster to the side, and stretch your legs.

VARIATION

A nice variation would be to place a Rectangle Fold blanket at the top of your bolster and rest your forehead on the blanket. The blanket leaves space for you to breathe, and also puts gentle pressure on your vagus nerve, which is very calming.

OPTION 2

WHAT TO DO

1. As an alternative, if your knees are not happy in Child's Pose, use two chairs facing each other corner to corner. Place the bolster on an angle on one chair seat and rest the upper end against the back of the chair. Sit on the corner of the second chair facing the bolster, and fold forward with your whole belly resting on the bolster. You may raise the bolster higher by using an additional bolster or by placing the bolster on an angle with one or two blocks at whatever height makes the bolster feel comfortable. Rest your arms where they are comfortable.

2. Turn your head to one side and rest your cheek on the bolster or your folded hands. Halfway through the pose, turn your head and rest on your other cheek for an equal length of time.

3. Stay in the posture for at least five minutes. When you are finished, gently uncurl your body, move the bolster to the side, and stretch your legs.

YOGIC WISDOM

If you are pregnant, you can still do Child's Pose. Just leave a little space for your belly and rest your chest and head on the bolster.

FAN POSE

Chakra Benefited:

Doshic Balance: K–, P+, V=

YOU NEED:

- Mat
- Blanket (Rectangle Fold) (optional)
- Bolster
- Blanket (Head Rest Fold or Rectangle Fold) (optional)
- Chair (optional)
- 2 blocks (optional)

Fan Pose is a relaxing forward bend that opens up your inner thighs and stretches the lower back. It helps quiet the organs, and get any stagnant energy in the legs moving again. Use this pose to direct your focus inward after a long, busy, stressful day.

WHAT TO DO

1. Sit on your mat facing the long side. Open your legs into a comfortable "fan" position. Your legs should be wide enough apart that you can feel a stretch, but not so far as to cause pain in your buttocks or behind your knees. If you have difficulty sitting straight up, sit on a blanket in the Rectangle Fold to tilt your hips forward.

2. Place the narrow end of a bolster between your legs. Fold forward from your hips and rest your belly on the bolster. Rest your forehead on the bolster, or turn your head to the side and rest your cheek on it. Use a blanket in the Head Rest Fold or Rectangle Fold underneath your head for added cushioning, if you want. Arms should rest on each side of the bolster, or can be draped over the bolster.

3. Hold this pose for at least five minutes. To come out of the pose, bring your torso upright, move the bolster, and bring your legs together.

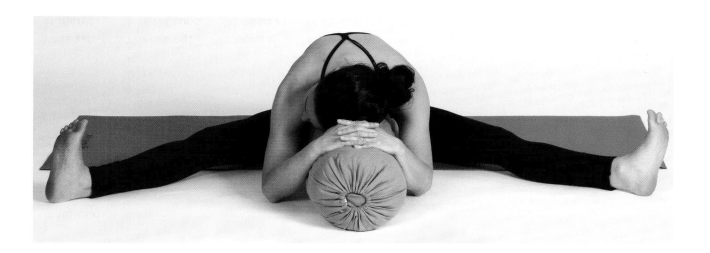

VARIATION

An alternative to this pose is to sit on the floor and rest your arms on a chair, with your legs on each side of the chair legs. However you choose to do this pose, remember that finding a comfortable bolster height is key. You don't want to overstretch your lower back. Experiment by raising the height of the bolster by placing a block or two underneath the head of the bolster, using more than one bolster, or using blankets in smaller increments to raise the prop closer to you. Your arms should be comfortable, too. If your arms don't touch the floor, prop them up with blankets, or rest them on the bolster.

BELLY DOWN WITH BOLSTER AT HIP

Chakras Benefited:

Doshic Balance: K+, P+, V–

YOU NEED:
- Mat
- Bolster

This pose is not truly a forward bend, but it has similar effects, which is why it's placed in this section. You can use this pose as a nice counterstretch to release any back tension. It's great for women's issues, such as menstrual cramps, as well.

WHAT TO DO

1. Lay a mat on the floor. Place the bolster across the middle of your mat.

2. Kneel at the bolster, facing the top end of your mat. Position your hips at the bolster, and lay your body forward over the top so that your hips are raised on it Bring your arms forward, elbows bent, and place one hand on top of the other. Lower your head and rest your forehead on your hands. Keep your legs and feet relaxed, with your feet resting on the floor so that your ankles turn out and your toes turn in.

3. Hold this position for at least five minutes. Focus on your breath while in the pose.

4. Press your hands into the floor and lift yourself back off the bolster. Go back to **Child's Pose Option 1**, but keep your arms draped over the bolster in their horizontal position for a few moments before you come out of the pose.

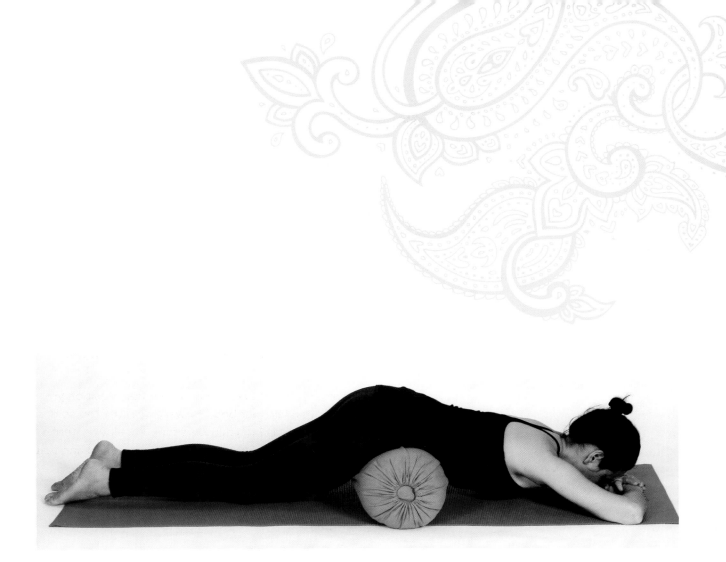

THREADS OF THOUGHT

Yogaś-citta-vrtti-nirodha

When you reach a state of yoga, your mind will find true tranquility. All of your changing emotions, perceptions of things, and judgments (citta vrtti) come to rest (nirodha).

CHAIR FORWARD BEND

FOR OPTION 1 YOU NEED:
- Mat
- Chair
- Blanket (Square Fold) (optional)
- Blanket (Rectangle Fold) (optional)
- 2 blocks (optional)

Chakras Benefited:

Doshic Balance: K+, P+, V–

All forward bends are calming to the mind, but it's hard to relax when you feel like you are overstretching! The beauty of this Chair Forward Bend is that you feel supported while holding the shape. Your body will stretch, but you won't feel like you've overdone it.

OPTION 1

WHAT TO DO

1. Place the chair at the top of your mat with the seat facing toward you. Sit in a cross-legged position in front of the chair. Fold forward so that your forearms are resting on the seat of the chair with your elbows bent. Rest your forehead on your forearms. You may place a Square Fold blanket on the seat of the chair to soften it, if you choose. You may also use a Rectangle Fold blanket under your buttocks for comfort. If needed, you can prop up your bent knees with blocks.

2. Hold the pose for at least three minutes before you switch the cross of your legs.

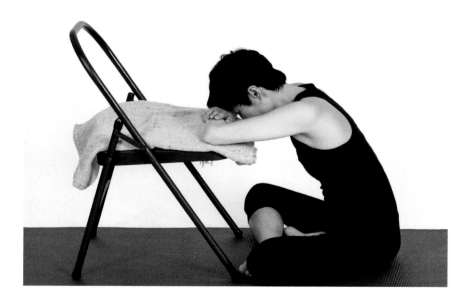

FOR OPTION 2 YOU NEED:
- Mat
- Chair
- Blanket (Square Fold) (optional)
- Blanket (Rectangle Fold) (optional)
- Blanket (Short Roll Fold) or block (optional)

OPTION 2

WHAT TO DO

1. Place the chair at the top end of your mat with the seat facing toward you. Sit in front of the chair with one leg out straight in front of you under the chair, and one knee bent, with the foot folded toward your pelvis. For an extra stretch, you can place the foot of your straight leg on the back rung of the chair. Fold forward so that your forearms are resting on the seat of the chair with your elbows bent. Rest your forehead on your forearms. If you cannot reach the seat of the chair with your head, pull the chair closer to you. You may place a Square Fold blanket on the seat of the chair to soften it, if you choose. You may also use a Rectangle Fold blanket under your buttocks for comfort. If needed, you can prop up your bent knee with a block or a Short Roll Fold blanket.

2. Hold the pose for at least three minutes before you switch the straight leg and bent leg.

VARIATIONS

For both options, the priority is being comfortable and not causing any strain to your lower back or knees. You can raise your buttocks on a blanket for more comfort in your back. If you feel any pressure on your knees, place rolled blankets or blocks underneath your knees for support.

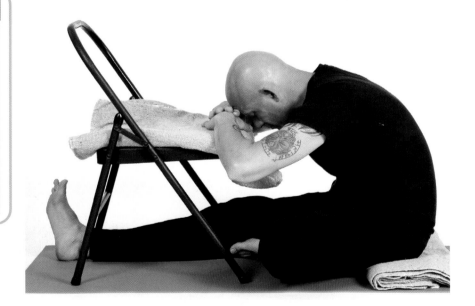

DOWN DOG WITH HEAD ON BLOCK OR BOLSTER

Chakras Benefited:

Doshic Balance: K+, P+, V–

YOU NEED:
- Mat
- Block or bolster

This forward bend is a staple in active yoga classes. It is an inversion that is very calming to the mind. With this supported version in restorative yoga, however, you don't put any strain on your neck. It creates a feeling of "letting go" while giving the diaphragm a rest, allowing you to release your breath, and loosening up tight shoulder muscles. It's also good for those with high blood pressure. Try it to relieve lower back pain.

WHAT TO DO

1. Place a mat on the floor, and your block or bolster lengthwise on it, at the top of the mat. Get onto your hands and knees, distributing your weight equally on all fours. Your hands should be underneath your shoulders, and your knees should be under your hips. (You can adjust the position of your hands and feet slightly once you get into the pose.)

2. Move the block or a bolster down the mat between your arms, to a position roughly underneath your breastbone.

3. Curl your toes under and lift your knees away from the ground. It's fine to keep your knees bent slightly. Your head and upper torso will pivot down in response to your knees and hips lifting.

4. Rest your forehead on the block or bolster. Adjust the height of your head support to avoid any strain in the neck. Try not to bend your elbows to get your head down to the support; it's better to adjust the height of prop. Rest here for at least one minute. As your legs stretch and open up, challenge yourself to straighten them more.

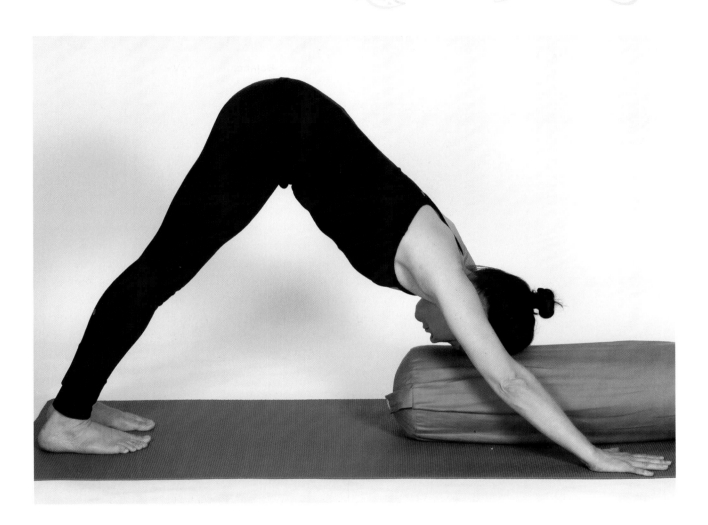

5. To come out of the pose, lower to your knees and rest for a few moments in **Child's Pose**. (Note: For this pose, **Child's Pose** will be done without any props. Just fold yourself over your legs.)

PIGEON POSE
WITH BOLSTER

YOU NEED:
- Mat
- Bolster
- Block (optional)
- 1–2 blankets (Rectangle Fold, Small Square Fold, or Oblong Fold)

Chakra Benefited:

Doshic Balance: K+, P+, V–

Almost everyone is in need of Pigeon Pose. If you sit in a chair or drive in a car for long periods of time—like most people do today—you likely have tension in your hips, which can cause all sorts of problems with the piriformis muscle and sciatic nerve pushing against each other in this tight, densely packed area of the body. In yoga, the hips are thought of as "closets" because they carry so much tension associated with our emotions, which makes them important areas to focus on in restorative yoga. In this supported version of Pigeon Pose, you use a bolster for added support to create a better sense of relaxation and release. Hold this pose for as long as you can to "clean out your closet."

WHAT TO DO

1. Place a mat on the floor. Place the bolster lengthwise along the center, toward the top of the mat. Begin in **Down Dog with Head on Block or Bolster** (without the block or bolster under your head).

2. Keeping your left toes curled against the floor, raise your right leg and bring your right knee up along your body toward your right wrist, then lower your hips down. Keep your hands alongside you to help you lengthen your spine.

3. Reach for the bolster and move it down the center of the mat, aligned with your spine and under your torso, and rest it against your right shin. Lay your belly down over the bolster. You can place your hands on the bolster and rest your forehead on your hands, or turn your head to one side and rest your cheek against the bolster with your arms resting on the floor alongside. You can raise the head of the bolster up on a block if it's more comfortable. Use a blanket or two in the Rectangle Fold or Small Square Fold under the hip above your bent knee if you find yourself leaning to that

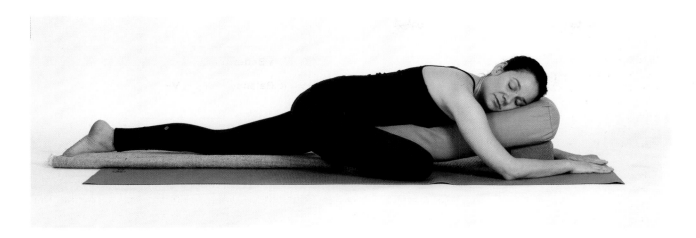

side. Relax your feet and allow the toes to uncurl once you have settled in. For more comfort on the back knee, place an Oblong Fold blanket under the back leg. Rest here for at least three minutes. If you are resting your cheek against the bolster, turn your head halfway through the pose to rest your other cheek against it.

4. Rise back up into **Down Dog with Head on Block or Bolster** (without the block or bolster). Jog out your legs, then repeat the pose on the left side.

VARIATION

*For more knee and hip support (especially if you suffer from knee issues), place the bolster underneath your thigh and across the mat, instead of in front of you aligned with the center of your torso. To do: From **Down Dog with Head on Block or Bolster**, lunge forward with one leg and place the bolster under your thigh. Bring your foot over to the opposite side, and lower down over the bolster. The bolster should be horizontal on your mat with the shin parallel to it, so the thigh rests on the bolster. Flex your toes to take any pressure off your knee. Fold forward so that your arms are on the floor, and rest your head on your hands out in front of you with your elbows bent.*

INVERSIONS

Most of our time is spent either standing up, sitting down, or lying down. We are rarely inverted, which is too bad, because there are many benefits to turning ourselves upside down once in a while. Fortunately, inversions are an integral part of most yoga sequences. According to Iyengar yoga, inversions and the "reversing gravity" effect they create can help to give your organs a rest and shift the fluids that have settled in your feet back up through your body, for an overall restorative benefit. During inversion poses, fresh lymphatic fluid flows through the body and fresh blood flows back to the heart and to the brain, improving the function of the immune system and fostering mental clarity. Other benefits from these poses include the release of lactic acid, which helps relieve tired legs or feet (great if you've overdone it at the gym); gentle stretching of the back of the legs; and relief of mild backaches. Inversions are also great for relieving jet lag! One of the most valuable benefits of inversions, however, is that they calm the mind, which is the heart of restorative yoga.

YOGIC WISDOM

The beauty of the inversions in restorative yoga is that they benefit almost everyone, and offer a safe alternative to the traditional poses. For example, Legs Up the Wall (both with and without bolster) is a safe alternative to the traditional headstand for someone with neck issues (such as stiffness or herniation), and Chair Shoulder Stand is safe for someone with shoulder issues. However, inversions, even in restorative yoga, are not recommended if you have problems with detached retinas, are suffering from serious heart problems, or are experiencing a severe headache.

LEGS UP THE WALL POSE WITHOUT BOLSTER

Chakra Benefited:

Doshic Balance: K–, P+, V=

Note: This is *not* recommended for women who are in the second and third trimesters of pregnancy, but it is a safe pose for those who have glaucoma.

YOU NEED:
- Mat
- Wall
- Blanket (Head Rest Fold) (optional)
- Blanket (Open Fold, to drape over your body) (optional)

This pose is similar to Legs Up the Wall Pose with Bolster, but it can be done anywhere you have a wall. Use this pose to gain a sense of calm and restoration after a long day, or after a tough workout to relieve your legs of any lactic acid. In yoga, inversions are not usually recommended for women who are menstruating, but this pose can be done during your cycle when it's not too heavy.

WHAT TO DO

1. Come onto your side on the floor and curl up in a fetal position, bringing your buttocks as close to the wall as possible.

2. Roll onto your back and stretch your legs up the wall. Keep your arms extended to the sides in a T- or U-shape. If you find your chin is tilted too far back and overextended, use a blanket in the Head Rest Fold under your head to bring it level with your chest.

3. For extra warmth, if desired, drape an open blanket over your feet. Settle in and connect to your breath. Hold this position for a minimum of five minutes, and as long as twenty.

4. To come out of the pose, bend your knees, and then roll to your right side to come up.

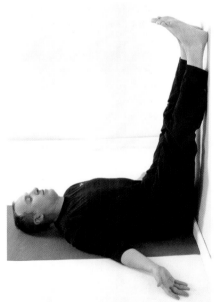

> ### VARIATION
>
> *Practice variations of this pose for a few minutes each if you want to stretch different parts of the legs: Legs in Fan Position; Legs in Bound Angle Pose; Legs in Cross-Legged Position (make sure to switch crosses and spend an equal time in each).*

LEGS UP THE WALL POSE WITH BOLSTER

Chakra Benefited:

Doshic Balance: K–, P+, V=

Note: This pose is not recommended if you are in the second and third trimesters of pregnancy, as lying flat on your back can be dangerous.

YOU NEED:

- Mat
- Block
- Wall
- 2 bolsters
- Blanket (Rectangle Fold) (optional)

This pose is a favorite of many, as it is a great overall restorative pose and has many of the physical benefits of a back bend. It reinvigorates tired legs and feet, calms the nervous system, and is great for rebalancing your energy while traveling, because it helps circulate your blood after you have been sitting for a while. It even helps reduce swelling in your legs, a common issue associated with air travel. The pose is relatively easy to do. It is said that twenty minutes spent in this pose has the same beneficial effect on your nervous system as taking a nap (but a waking nap—stay connected to your breath!), because the benefit of the pose has the same effect on your nervous system. The pose has many of the physical benefits of a back bend, because it can be so rejuvenating.

WHAT TO DO

1. Place a block on the short height with the long side against the wall, and then place a bolster with the long side against the block. Remove the block (it's just a space measurement for the bolster).

2. If desired, take a Rectangle Fold blanket and drape it over the middle of the bolster so that it forms a T-shape over the middle of the bolster. The remainder of the blanket should sit on your mat.

3. Sit sideways, one hip against the bolster, and lower your shoulder and head to the floor beside you.

4. Roll onto your back, stretch your legs up the wall, and reposition yourself until your tailbone is tilted up over the bolster.

5. Extend your arms to the sides in a T- or U-shape. If necessary, support your neck by rolling up the Rectangle Fold blanket that is in the middle of your mat.

VARIATION

If you have tight hamstrings, you may want more of a bend in your knees. Practice this pose with your lower back resting on the bolster and your legs slightly away from the wall, with a second bolster resting vertically up the wall to support your thighs. You can also put a Long Roll Fold blanket behind your knees for extra support.

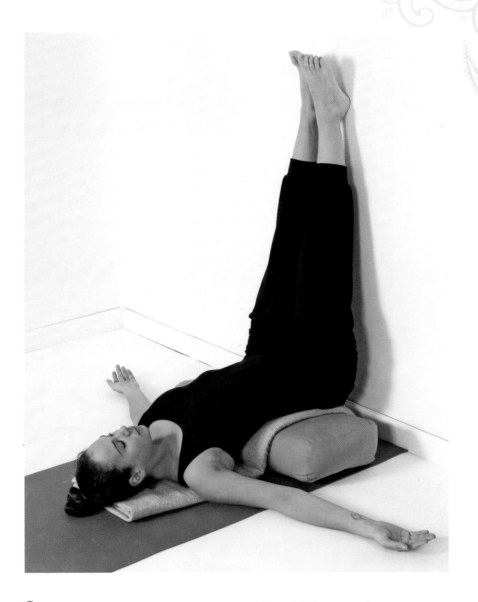

6. Settle in and connect to your breath. Hold this pose for a minimum of five minutes, and for a maximum of twenty.

7. To come out of this pose, bend your knees, push the bolster toward the wall, and then roll to your right side to come up.

LEGS ON CHAIR

Chakra Benefited:

Doshic Balance: K–, P+, V=

The hamstrings can become an issue in inversions—if they are tight, raising the legs straight up can strain the hamstrings, making the pose uncomfortable. The beauty of this pose is that the chair supports the calves, which puts the hamstrings at ease. You get the benefits of an inversion—including a calmed nervous system, restored legs and feet, and a relaxed lower back—without any of the discomfort. *Note:* This pose is not recommended for pregnant women in their third trimester.

YOU NEED
- Mat
- Chair
- Blanket (Square Fold)
  Blanket (Head Rest Fold)
- Bolster (optional)

WHAT TO DO

1. Place the chair on your yoga mat.

2. Place a Square Fold blanket on the seat of the chair.

3. Lie on one side and roll onto your back, placing your calves on the seat of the chair. Do not let the back of your knees touch the edge of the chair seat.

4. Place your arms in either a T- or U-shape position or alongside your body with space between your body and arms. Support your neck with a blanket in the Head Rest Fold, if desired. If you wish to use a bolster under your lower back, press your calves into the seat of the chair to lift your hips up, and slide the bolster underneath your lower back.

5. Settle in and connect to your breath. Hold this position for a minimum of five minutes, and for as long as twenty minutes.

6. To come out of this pose, bend your knees and hug them in toward you, and roll to your right side to come up.

THREADS OF THOUGHT

Heyaṁ dukham-anāgatam

Past and present suffering cannot be avoided; they are the fruits of our karma. But future suffering can be avoided, through the practice of yoga.

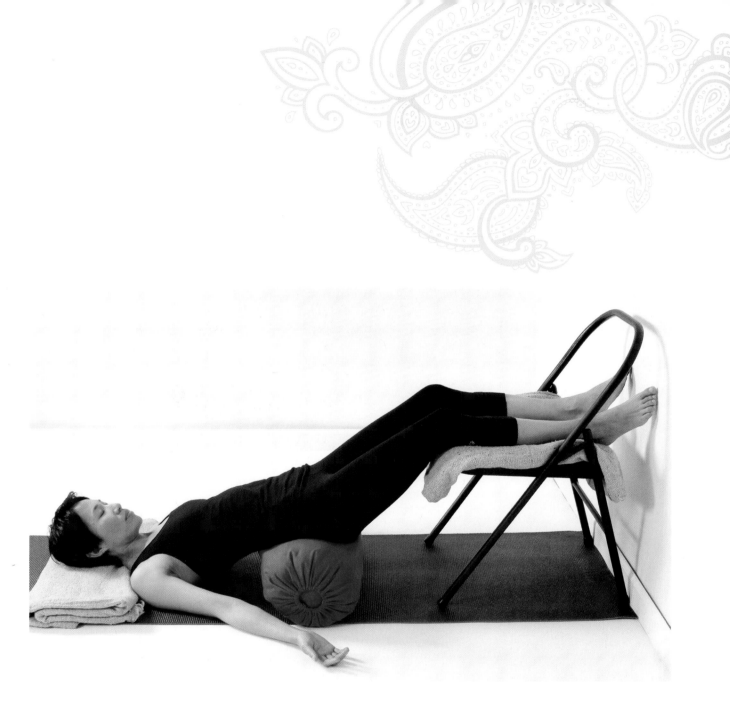

TWO CHAIR BOAT POSE

Chakra Benefited:

Doshic Balance: K–, P+, V=

YOU NEED:

- Mat
- Blanket (Square Fold)
- 2 chairs
- 6 blocks
- 2 bolsters
- 2 blankets (Square Fold) (optional)
- Blanket (Head Rest Fold) (optional)
- Blanket (Open Fold, to drape over you) (optional)

This pose requires a bit more effort to set up, but don't be discouraged—it is worth it. This a very calming pose that helps restore the nervous system, and it can also help relieve any emotional trauma if you drape a blanket over you for a quieting cocoon effect. Usually inversions are not recommended for women who are past their first trimester of pregnancy, but this one is safe.

WHAT TO DO

1. Place a Square Fold blanket on your mat for extra padding.

2. Place both chairs upside down on the mat so that the legs face each other. The Square Fold blanket should be between them.

3. Place 2 blocks on the short height on the underside of each chair seat. Lean a bolster along the blocks on each chair seat, one narrow end resting on the Square Fold blanket. (The blocks are there to support the bolster, so it doesn't sag.) It should look like a V-shape when you are done setting up.

4. Bring your body between the chairs and lay your back on one bolster/chair setup. Lift your legs up to rest on the other bolster/chair setup. Adjust the distance between the chairs until you are comfortable and don't feel any strain on your back or legs. Drape a Square Fold blanket over each leg of the chair by your torso for extra padding against your shoulders, if you like. If you need support for your head, place a Head Rest Fold blanket under your head. For an added "cocoon" feeling, drape a blanket over the entire setup like a tent, so you feel completely enclosed and safe.

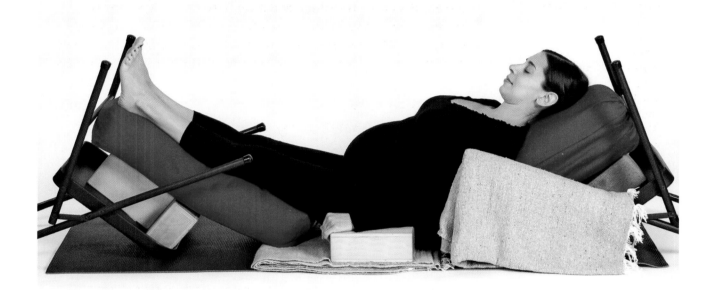

5. Rest your forearms on your torso or on the remaining two blocks. Settle in and connect to your breath. Hold this position for a minimum of five minutes, and for as long as twenty.

6. To come out of this pose, set your feet against the far chair and straighten your legs so that the chair is pushed away from you. Bend your knees, and roll to your right side to come out.

CHAIR SHOULDER STAND

Chakra Benefited:

Doshic Balance: K–, P+, V=

YOU NEED:
- Mat
- Chair
- Blanket (Square Fold)
- Bolster
- Wall
- Blanket (Rectangle Fold) (optional)

This pose gives you the benefits of a shoulder stand, considered to be the mother of all poses. It soothes your nerves, relieves insomnia, improves digestion, lessens the strain on your heart, helps relieve the common cold by alleviating nasal congestion via increasing blood flow to the head, and benefits your immune system. All this without the anxiety that comes from doing it without support! It's challenging, but worth the effort.

WHAT TO DO

1. Place a chair on your yoga mat, seat facing you, slightly away from the wall. Place a Square Fold blanket on the seat of the chair. Then place a bolster on the mat, the long side against the front of the chair.

2. Sit facing the wall on the chair, straddling the chair. Begin to swing your legs up over the chair to rest on the wall. As you raise your legs, start to lower your back down over the chair. Using your arms to help brace yourself, slide your upper body down toward the bolster on the floor, leaving only your lower back resting on the chair. Your shoulders will rest on the bolster. If desired, use a Rectangle Fold blanket to support your head. Your arms may be in a T- or U-shape or whatever feels most comfortable to you. Rest here for five to fifteen minutes.

3. Next, lower yourself further down, so that your lower back is resting on the bolster and your torso is lying on the floor. Try to drop your tailbone toward the floor slightly. Allow your legs to form a diamond shape with the knees bent and the feet toward each other while they rest on the seat of the chair. Rest here for a minimum of five minutes and a maximum of twenty, unless you are ready to come out the pose entirely (if so, hold this second pose for only one minute).

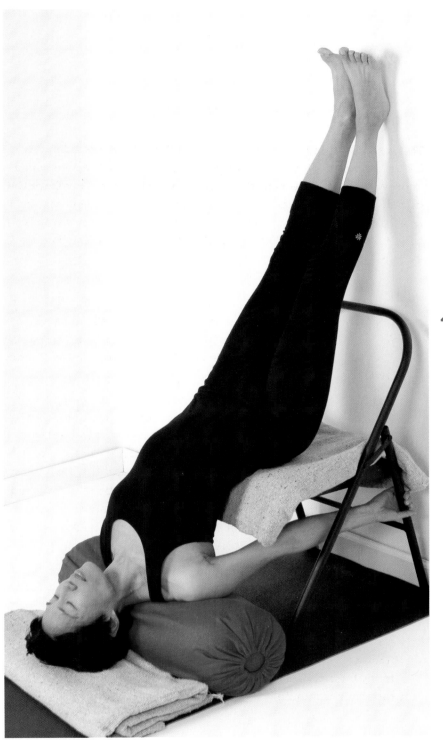

4. To come out of the pose, push yourself away from the chair, sliding your buttocks off the bolster so that your lower back is resting on the floor. Then you can roll to your side, rest for a moment, and press yourself up to a sitting position.

> **YOGIC WISDOM**
>
> *Make sure your neck is fully supported in this pose. You don't want it jammed toward your chest, or overextended in any way. Use a Rectangle Fold Blanket under your head for added support, if needed.*

POSES OF COMPLETION

Savasana (pronounced sha-vah-sah-nah) is the pose that seals it all in. The word *savasana* means "corpse" in Sanskrit. The idea behind this posture is that in it, we learn to "die." This may sound morbid, but when you practice the pose properly, you begin to understand the importance of this idea. On an emotional level, savasana helps you learn to let go, or "die" to the things that hold you emotionally and physically locked. And the art of letting go is at the heart of restorative yoga.

The poses of completion in this section help the body to integrate all the poses performed before it, so these poses should always be done at the end of your practice. However, the poses are not meant for you to fall asleep in, and herein lies the challenge, as they're so relaxing! Savasana poses should be held for a minimum of ten minutes, but it really takes a good fifteen minutes to really go deep. Try to "witness" yourself in Savasana; observe yourself as you are relaxed and awake. There are many variations of Savasana, and specific variations are best for emotional issues like trauma or abuse, while others are best for pregnancy or injury.

THREADS OF THOUGHT

Tadā drashtu svarūpe-'vasthānam

Imagine yourself as the sea: only when you can see through the shifting water (citta vrtti; your changing thoughts and emotions) to the bottom, can you find your true self (drashtu).

PRONE (ON BELLY) SAVASANA

YOU NEED:
- Mat
- Bolster (optional)

Chakras Benefited:

Doshic Balance: K+, P−, V=

This version of Savasana promotes an inward focus, and is good for anyone looking for an emotionally soothing pose. Closing off the front body makes you feel nurtured and safe, especially if you have suffered trauma. This pose is a good therapy for a particularly hard day. You can use a variety of props for this pose. Before beginning, set up any props you want to use. As an example, you may choose to use a Rectangle Fold blanket under your head, or a Long Roll Fold blanket under the tops of your feet.

WHAT TO DO

1. Instead of lying down on your back as you would for traditional Savasana, lie down on your belly. Let your feet turn in toward each other. If desired, you can lay a bolster across on your mat, and lay your pelvic bones over the bolster as you lie down onto your belly.

2. Bend your arms at the elbows, placing one hand on the other, palms down. Rest your forehead on your hands. You may also turn your head to one side and then switch to the other side for an equal amount of time.

3. Relax here for as long as you feel comfortable. To come out, press back onto your heels and rest for a moment in **Child's Pose Option 1**.

VARIATION

If you have intestinal issues like constipation or menstrual cramps, take a blanket, roll it up in a tight ball, tuck it against the soft part of your belly under your ribs, and lie down on it. Rest for as long as you feel comfortable. Try to take deep abdominal breaths while in this pose. When you come out of the pose, press back onto your heels and rest for a moment in **Child's Pose Option 1**.

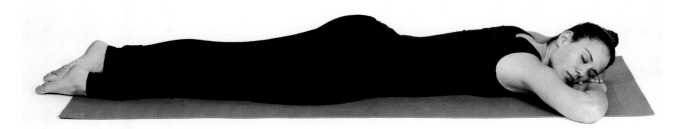

SAVASANA

Chakras Benefited: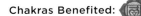

Doshic Balance: K+, P–, V=

At its most basic level, Savasana can be done with no props at all. That being said, the premise of restorative yoga is to feel supported, so it's good to use any and all props that help you feel supported in the pose.

YOU NEED:

- Mat
- Blanket (Head Rest Fold) (optional)
- Bolster (optional)
- 1–3 blankets (Long Roll Fold) (optional)
- Blanket (Open Fold)(optional)
- 1–2 sandbags (optional)
- Eye pillow or headwrap (optional)

WHAT TO DO

1. Lie comfortably on a mat. Hug one knee into your chest, then lower your leg down to lie along the floor. Hug the other knee into your chest, then lower that leg down to lie along the floor. Stretch out your arms to create space in your armpits. Your hands may lie palms up, or on the sides of the hands with the palms facing your body.

2. Do a quiet scan of your body and determine if and how you need to use the props for comfort. Where do you need extra support? Bring your hands behind your head with your elbows bent to draw your chin in toward your chest. Then, slowly lower your head down toward the floor as you work to elongate your neck. If your neck is still not comfortable as you lower your head down, place a blanket in the Head Rest Fold under your head. Next, check in with your lower back. If it is not comfortable, place a bolster underneath your slightly bent knees. Resting your feet on a blanket in the Long Roll Fold, placed under the Achilles tendons, can be very beneficial as well. For additional weight and relaxation, drape an open blanket on top of you, and/or place sandbags on your shoulders or your abdomen. Use an eye pillow or headwrap, if you like. Use a blanket in the Long Roll Fold along the outside of each arm for support. Using these props to support your body helps promote deep relaxation.

YOGIC WISDOM

If you have a headache, some helpful tools for this pose are a block and a sandbag. Place the block behind your head on the floor with a sandbag propped on it, and partially resting on your forehead. Be mindful while moving the props, so that you don't strain yourself.

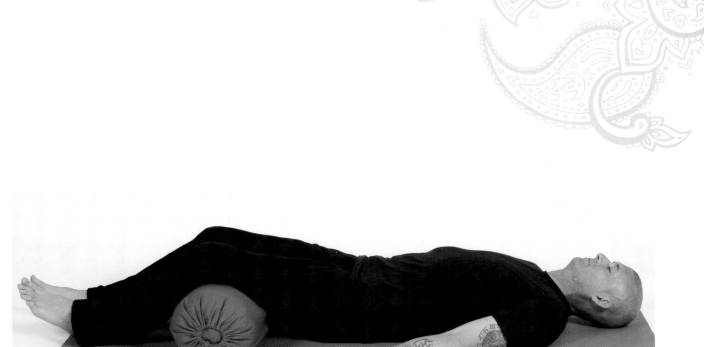

3. To come out of this pose, begin to move the parts of your body in micro movements, by wiggling your fingers and toes. Then you can slowly hug your knees into your chest, and roll to your right side (unless you are pregnant, in which case roll to your left) to adjust. Press up to a sitting position from there.

SIDE LYING SAVASANA

Chakras Benefited:

Doshic Balance: K+, P−, V=

YOU NEED:
- Mat
- 2 blankets (Small Square Fold)
- 2–3 bolsters
- Blanket (Open Fold) (optional)

Side Lying Savasana, a heavily supported version of Savasana, is for everyone. It is especially effective at relieving fatigue and high blood pressure, and is a good version to use when you are experiencing indigestion or stomach upset, as it relieves discomfort and stimulates digestion. Pregnant women find this version effective during the last months of their pregnancy, when they are in most need of relief from the weight they are carrying, and it is the safest because it does not put pressure on the inferior vena cava (the large vein that returns blood from the lower half of the body to the heart). Lying on your back in pregnancy causes the uterus to put pressure on the inferior vena cava, which can make feel like you are going to pass out or feel nauseated.

WHAT TO DO

1. Lie down on your left side and bring your left arm out away from you.

2. Place a Small Square Fold blanket under your head.

3. Place one bolster from your knee to your ankle between your legs. Place another bolster in front of your belly, so that your top arm can drape over the bolster. Adjust for comfort with an additional Small Square Fold blanket under your ankles so that your knee and ankle are on the same level. You may choose to put an additional bolster behind your back for a feeling of being more supported, so you can relax deeper. Place a blanket over you, if desired. Hold this position for a minimum of ten minutes and a maximum of twenty minutes, to get the true benefits of this pose.

VARIATION

If you'd like, you can use the wall for back support in this pose. Set up with your mat against the wall lengthwise. If you want the wall for support against your back, place a bolster lengthwise against the wall, parallel with your mat. Use a Small Square Fold blanket under your head for support.

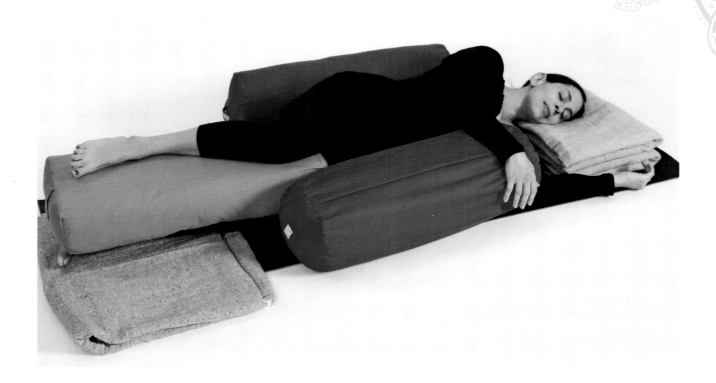

4. To come out of this pose, remove the props between your legs and in front of you. Slowly press up to a sitting position, with your head coming up last. Give yourself a few moments before getting up.

PART 3

THE SEQUENCES

*"At any moment, you have a choice, that either leads you
closer to your spirit or further away from it."*

—Thich Nhat Hanh, Vietnamese Zen Buddhist monk, teacher,
author, poet, and peace activist

This book has been set up to help you take your well-being into your own hands. You have been provided with enough information to experiment with, and see what works well for your particular body. No two people are exactly alike, and we all have had different experiences that have brought us to where we are today.

That being said, sometimes it is nice to be given a "lesson plan" that shows you a sequence with which to work to attain the maximum possible benefit. Restorative yoga is very purposeful; we don't approach chosen postures lightly. When you work with a yoga teacher or yoga therapist, he or she will set up a sequence that is geared toward your particular circumstance. Often the sequence will be repeated regularly, and will be adjusted and changed as needed.

In the pages that follow, you will find sequences of poses that reduce pain and help heal physical injury. Restorative yoga is for everyone: the most agile athlete, the injured person who is less (or not at all) athletic, the individual who wants to become more active, someone who has gotten out of practice in physical exercise, and someone who is healing from pain in parts of his or her body. In this chapter you will also find stress-reducing sequences, and sequences that help with emotional issues that you may deal with at certain times of your life, as well as progressions that are beneficial to your overall health.

For each ailment or issue found in this section, you can explore two options on how to find balance using restorative yoga:

- **Short Session:** Thirty minutes of three to four poses, to deepen your relaxation and open you to the benefit of the poses.

- **Long Session:** One to three hours, to help you really get into the mode of deep relaxation. This is where the major benefits of this practice kick in big time!

The sequences that follow cover specific issues and annoyances, and are just a small representation of what is possible in your healing. I know that you will find them helpful to you on your path to wellness.

Note: Throughout this section, you'll find a list of props needed to complete each particular sequence. Since the folds used for the blankets in each pose differ, you'll find information on both the overall number of blankets you'll need to complete a particular sequence, as well as the specific folds used throughout that sequence. Sometimes, you'll only need two blankets, but you'll find a variety of different folds listed for your convenience.

CHAPTER 6

THE SEQUENCES

"Yoga teaches us to cure what need not be endured and endure what cannot be cured."

—B.K.S. Iyengar, founder of Iyengar yoga, yoga master

The sequences in this chapter are based on therapy for physical and emotional ailments or issues. In many cases, the sequence provided for one issue will also be good for another, and a sidebar will call that out to you. A short sequence and a long sequence are given for each issue, enabling you to choose based on the time available to you on any given day. The short sequence should take about thirty minutes, and the long sequence can take an average of two hours.

Each pose in a sequence can be held for its minimum or maximum time, as noted in that pose's entry in Part 2. Decide how long to hold your pose based on the amount of time you have available to you, and also by how you feel in the pose. You may become uncomfortable after holding a pose for a while, which just means that you need to build up to holding it longer with comfort. In the meantime, come out of the pose when you feel uncomfortable.

Sometimes a pose in the sequence may not work for you. If this is the case, feel free to swap it out with another pose of its type, though each pose in the sequence has been chosen because it has a certain physiological or emotional effect. Also, please remember that you should be as comfortable as possible when holding a pose, so if you need to use additional props—even if they aren't called for in the pose instructions—by all means, use them. Restorative yoga is all about comfort, so make sure that this is what you're feeling as you work your way through the sequences found in this chapter.

SEQUENCES FOR THE UPPER BODY

The sequences in this section address stiffness in the upper body, which is one of the most common problem areas. Most people have neck, upper back, or shoulder issues at some point in their lives. The arms are an extension of the upper part of the body, and if you are misaligned there, you may find that you have issues in your arms, wrists, or elbows. The beauty of restorative yoga is that you can practice it despite acute or chronic pain, or even weaknesses in these areas. The passive poses help to promote better postural alignment, and they help you heal the areas affected. These sequences also help with recovery from surgery or injury in any of these areas. Please note that you should proceed with caution if you have had surgery, and make sure a doctor has cleared you to begin a physical activity before you begin.

NECK, UPPER BACK, SHOULDER, AND ARMS

TIME: 15–30 minutes

YOU NEED:
- Mat
- 2 blankets (Head Rest Fold and Long Roll Fold)
- 2 bolsters
- 2 blocks
- Chair (optional)
- 2 sandbags (or 2 bags of rice)
- Eye pillow (optional)

The neck in particular is very precarious when it comes to the slightest injury or tension. If your cervical vertebrae and their discs are misaligned, you may experience pain all the way down your arms to your fingertips. Your arms may have overall fatigue, or you may be suffering from tennis elbow or carpal tunnel syndrome. If you can learn to relax and let go of tension in these areas, the radiating pain that you experience will dissipate. Shoulders also hold a lot of tension, and as one of the weakest joints in the body they are prone to injury. If you work at a desk or do a lot of driving, you may feel upper back pain. Both of the restorative yoga sequences found here are great for relieving this strain.

SHORT SEQUENCE

WHAT TO DO

1. Begin by practicing **Neck Stretches**. Make sure you hold the stretch on each side for at least a couple of breaths, and lengthen it if you can by stretching your arms toward the floor—you want to really feel a full release in your neck area.

2. Next do **Eagle Arms**, making sure to take the time to drop your chin down and breathe a couple of times to really release the neck tension, and then finish the pose with your head lifted.

3. Now, move into the **Blanket Roll in 3 Positions (Position 1)**. Keep the blanket directly under your shoulder blades to get the full upper back stretch. Stay here for a minimum of two minutes. Roll to your right side as you come out, and then sit up and set up for your next pose.

4. Begin to concentrate on bringing fresh, restorative energy to your body by practicing **Heart Opening Pose**. Breathe deeply and feel the tension drift out of your body. Stay here for five minutes or more.

YOGIC WISDOM

If, at any time during this sequence, you feel uncomfortable (especially during Heart Opening Pose), feel free to add or remove any props. You need to be as comfortable as possible to reap the benefits of this and any sequence found throughout Part 3.

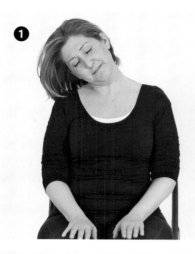

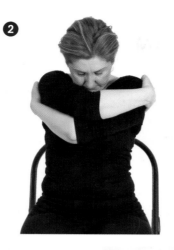

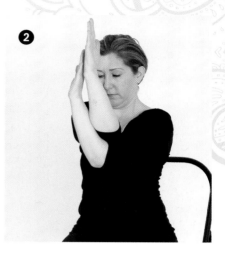

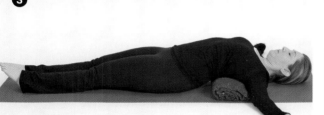

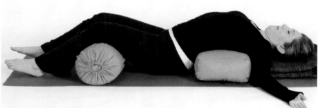

5. Place one bolster across the middle of your mat, and the other between your knees and feet to keep your pelvis supported for **Revolved Abdomen Pose**. Remember to hold the twist position for at least three minutes on each side.

6. Finish the sequence with **Savasana**. For this particular sequence, place one sandbag on each of your shoulders to help dispel any lingering tension there. Enjoy the extra weight on your shoulders, as you are sure to feel lighter after you remove them when Savasana is over. To really get the most out of this pose, hold it for a minimum of ten minutes.

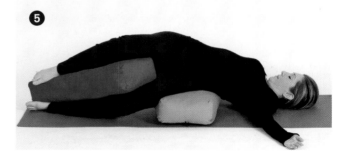

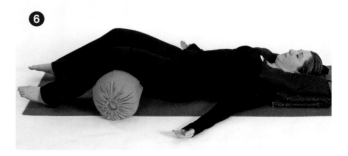

TIME: 45 minutes–2 hours

YOU NEED:
- Mat
- Wall
- 2 blankets (Head Rest Fold and Long Roll Fold)
- Strap/2 bolsters
- 2 blocks
- Chair (optional)
- 2 sandbags (or 2 bags of rice)
- Eye pillow (optional)

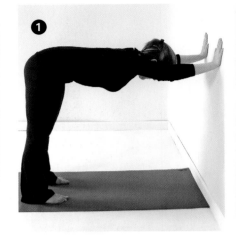
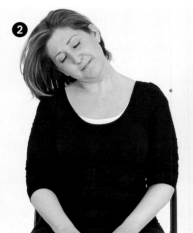
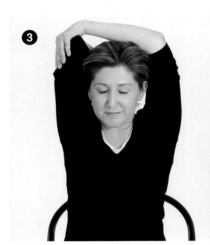
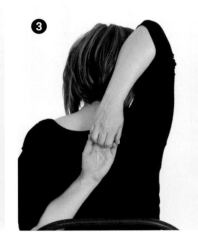
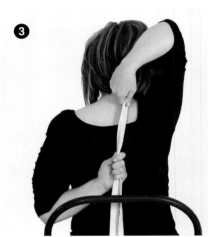

WHAT TO DO

1. Come to the wall for **Wall Downward-Facing Dog**. Concentrate on releasing the neck and shoulders with each exhale.

2. Do two rounds of **Neck Stretches** next.

3. From here do **Cow Face** pose on each side. Try to take at least three breaths on each side.

4. Continue with two rounds of **Shoulder Stretches**. Visualize releasing every muscle fiber in the upper body here.

5. Now move into the **Blanket Roll in 3 Positions (Position 1)**. Keep the blanket directly under your shoulder blades to get the full upper back stretch. Stay here for a minimum of two minutes.

6. Set up for **Heart Opening Pose**. Focus on opening the chest to release tension in the back for ten minutes.

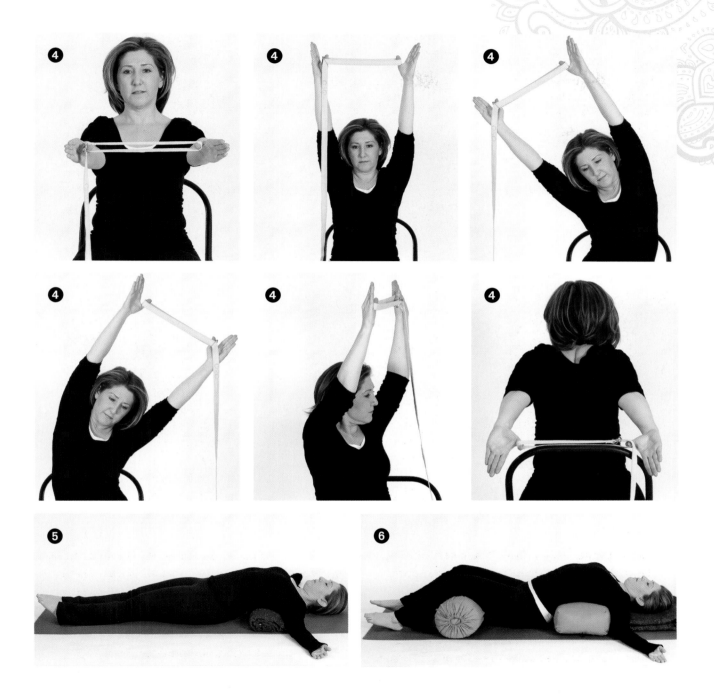

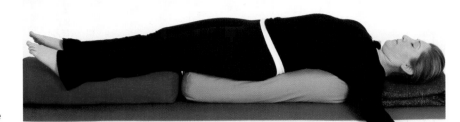

7. Next, set up for **Reclining Bridge Pose (Option 1)**. Again, focus on opening the chest here, stay for a minimum of eight minutes and a maximum of twenty.

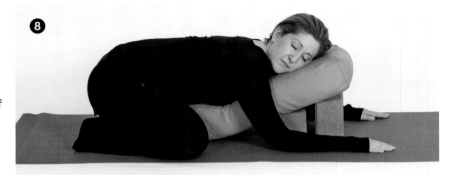

8. Come back into **Child's Pose (Option 1)**. Prolong your exhale to release tension, remain here for a minimum of six minutes and a maximum of fifteen.

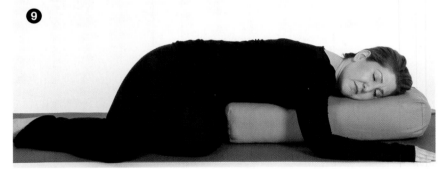

9. Set up for **Belly Down Twist over Bolster**. Here you want to concentrate on deepening the twist with every exhalation, to release tension in the upper body. Remain here for three minutes on each side.

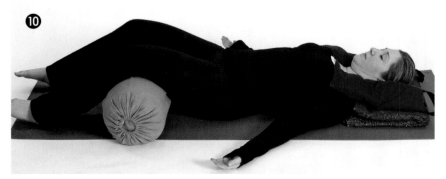

10. Finish the sequence with **Savasana**. For this particular sequence, place one sandbag on each of your shoulders to help dispel any lingering tension there. Enjoy the extra weight on your shoulders, as you are sure to feel lighter after you remove them when Savasana is over. To really get the most out of this pose, hold for a minimum of ten minutes.

SEQUENCES FOR THE LOWER BODY

From too much sitting, too much standing, wearing the wrong shoes, to working out too hard, the lower half of your body takes a beating. Whether you have a structural imbalance, an injury, or something hurting from repetitive stress, the following sequences will help you to find mobility in your lower body, as well as help relieve any pain you may be experiencing.

LEGS, KNEES, FEET

The legs, knees, and feet do a lot of work every day, which makes problems in these areas common. Your feet are probably the most ignored part of your body, but they bear all of your weight every day, and the way you walk can affect your legs. These sequences are geared toward tired legs and feet, and will also help relieve any knee discomfort. If you've recently had surgery on your legs, knees, or feet, these sequences should aid in your healing. However, remember to always remain comfortable and to come out of the pose the moment you begin to feel pain.

TIME: 40 minutes

YOU NEED:
- Mat
- Wall
- 2 blocks
- 2 straps
- 2 blankets
- Bolster
- Eye pillow (optional)

SHORT SEQUENCE

WHAT TO DO

1. Begin by coming into **Wall Half-Triangle Forward Bend** using a block underneath the ball of your forward foot. Hold this pose for two minutes on each side.

2. Next, transition into **Extended Hand to Foot Pose, Supine**. Hold one leg straight up, then out to the side, then across your body for one minute each. Switch to the other leg and repeat.

3. Move to the wall for **Legs Up the Wall Pose Without Bolster**. For this sequence, you need to strap your legs tightly in two places: one by the calf and one by the thighs. Hold for ten minutes, or less if you feel you need to come out sooner. Before you come out of the pose, remove the straps from your legs.

4. Transition into **Supported Bound Angle Pose (Option 2)** and hold for four minutes.

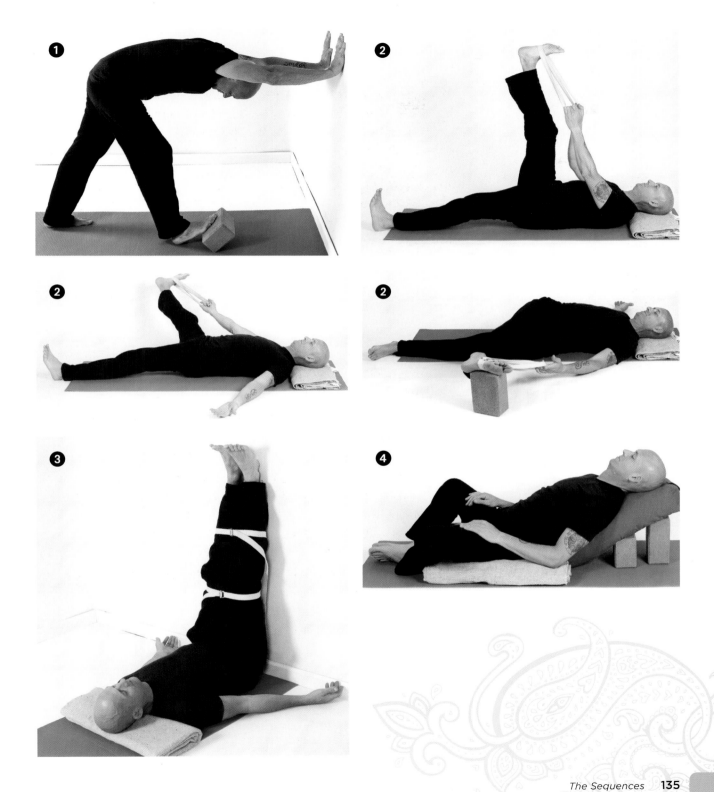

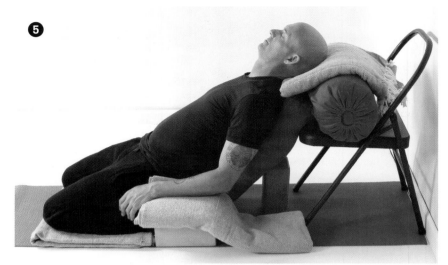

5. Set up for **Reclining Hero Pose (Option 3)** and hold for four minutes. Be sure to have a blanket under your shins and sit on a block to help relieve discomfort in your knees or feet.

6. Move into **Savasana**. Place a bolster underneath your knees and hold the pose for ten minutes. Use the eye pillow, if desired.

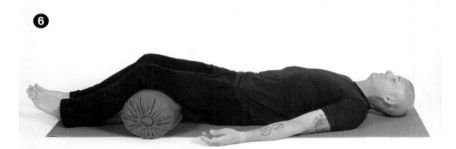

THREADS OF THOUGHT

Atha yoga-anuśāsanam

Your yoga practice begins wherever you are right now—tired, weak, energetic, or strong—yoga is ready when you are.

TIME: 1 hour

YOU NEED:
- Mat
- 2 blocks
- 2 straps
- Eye pillow (optional)
- Wall
- 2 blankets
- 2 bolsters
- Chair

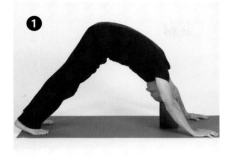

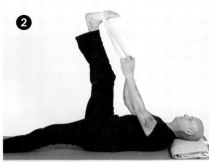

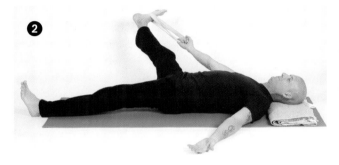

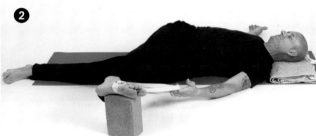

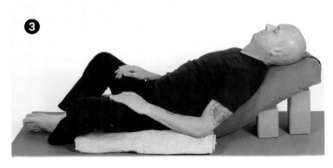

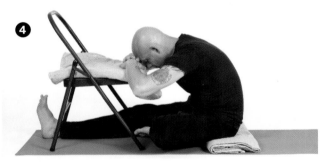

WHAT TO DO

1. Move into **Down Dog with Head on Block or Bolster**, using a block. Hold for three minutes.

2. Next, transition into **Extended Hand to Foot Pose, Supine**. Hold one leg straight up, then out to the side, then across your body for one minute each. Switch to the other leg and repeat.

3. Set up for **Supported Bound Angle Pose (Option 2)**. Hold for ten minutes.

4. Move to a chair for **Chair Forward Bend (Option 2)**. Hold for four minutes on each leg.

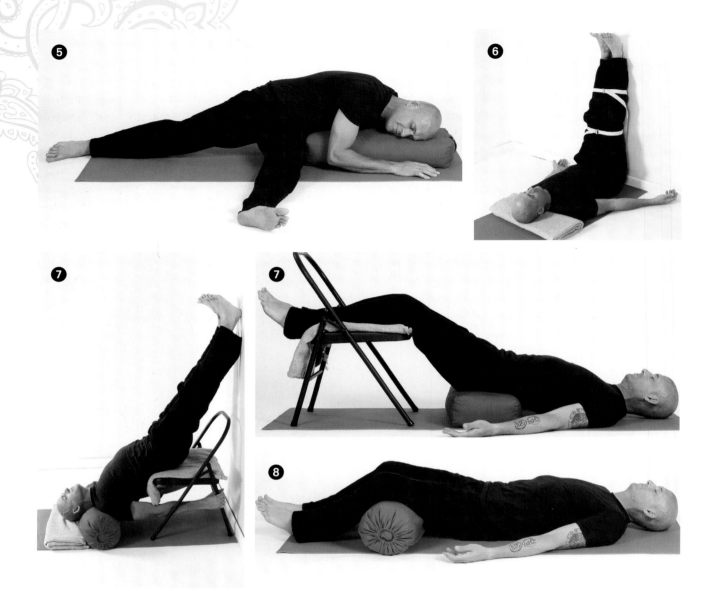

5. Move onto **Scissored Legs Belly Down Twist** and hold the position for three minutes on each side.

6. Move to the wall for **Legs Up the Wall Pose Without Bolster**. For this sequence, you need to strap your legs tightly in two places: one by the calf and one by the thighs (strap tightly). Hold for ten minutes.

7. Set up your chair for **Chair Shoulder Stand** and hold for six minutes. To come down from this pose, rest your lower back on the bolster and rest your legs on the seat of the chair for two or three minutes.

8. Finally, move to the floor for **Savasana**. Place a bolster under your knees and hold for twelve minutes. Use the eye pillow, if desired.

HIPS

TIME: 30 minutes

YOU NEED:
- Mat
- Strap
- 2 bolsters
- 2 blocks
- Blanket (Head Rest Fold) (optional)

As mentioned earlier, hips are known as the closets of your body because you hold or store a lot of tension in this area. It's important to understand that muscles have memory, and the memories you store in your hip area are related to feeling safe and secure. If you have had any experiences in your life that have compromised that feeling, you may have the tension of that experience release during your yoga practice. Tight hips can be the origin of problems all over your body, from your back all the way down to your knees. In Western society, we experience tight hips from sitting in chairs and cars for so much of our day. The following sequences will help your hips to feel more at ease, which will in turn help you feel more ease in your emotional life.

SHORT SEQUENCE

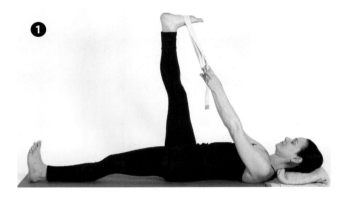

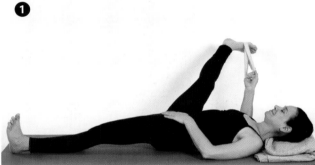

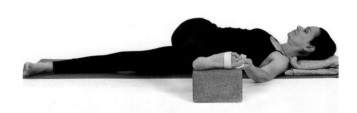

WHAT TO DO

1. Begin with **Extended Hand to Foot Pose, Supine**. While lying on your back, hold each leg up, out to the side, and across your body for one minute each before switching legs.

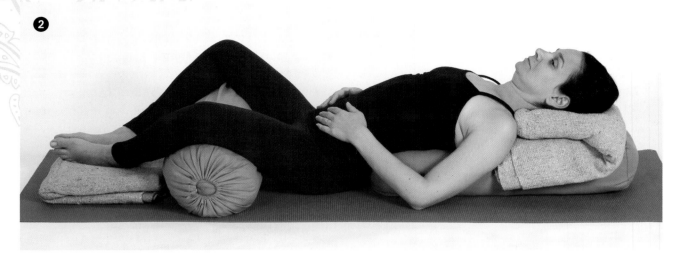

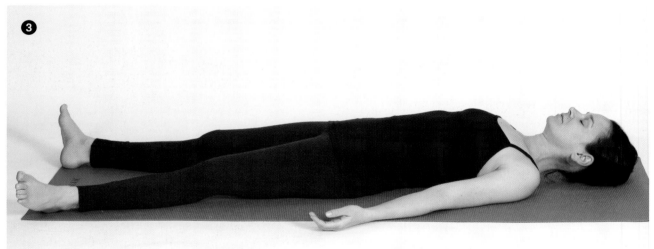

2. Set up for **Supported Bound Angle Pose (Option 4)**. For this sequence, place a bolster behind you—as shown in **Supported Bound Angle Pose (Option 1)**—and place another bolster underneath your knees, letting your legs open and your knees drop out to the sides. Hold for at least ten minutes.

3. Finish with **Savasana**. Lie on your back and rest fully for a minimum of five minutes and a maximum of fifteen minutes.

TIME: 1 hour

YOU NEED:
- Mat
- Strap
- 2 bolsters
- 2 blocks
- Blanket (Oblong Fold)
- Blanket (Head Rest Fold) (optional)

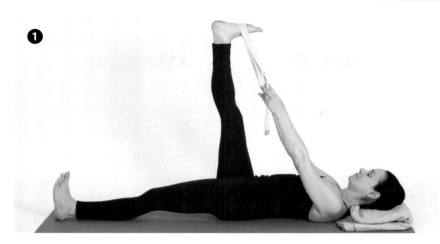

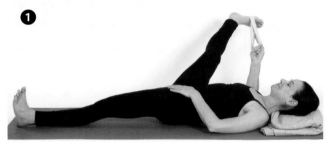

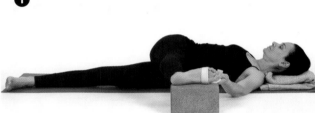

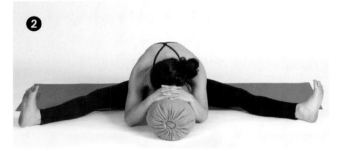

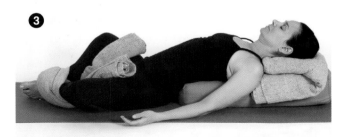

WHAT TO DO

1. Begin with **Extended Hand to Foot Pose, Supine**. While lying on your back, hold each leg up, out the side, and across your body for one minute each before switching legs.

2. Move on to **Fan Pose**. For this particular sequence, you will need one bolster. Hold each side for three minutes. If you prefer, you can place your head center, and rest your forehead on your hands.

3. Next move into **Supported Bound Angle Pose (Option 5)**. Rest in the pose for ten minutes.

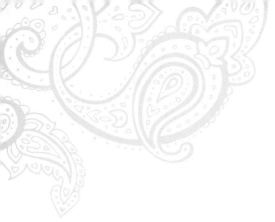

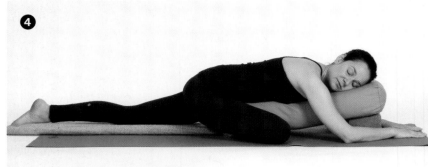

4. Continue to open your hips with **Pigeon Pose with Bolster**. Hold for three minutes on each side. Try to let yourself be supported by the bolster so you can relax as best you can.

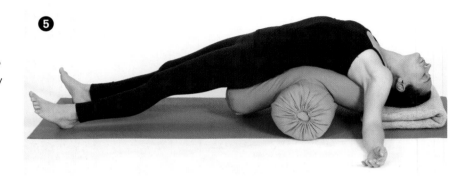

5. Next set up for **Cross Bolster Pose**. For this sequence, fully extend your legs: Lie back, and allow your front body to fully open. Hold for a minimum of four minutes.

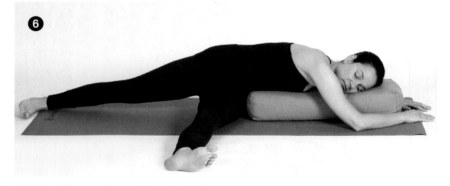

6. Come into **Scissored Legs Belly Down Twist**. Remember to lengthen your spine before you twist. Rest on each side for two minutes.

7. Finally, come into **Savasana**. Hold for ten minutes.

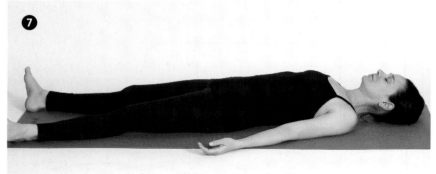

SEQUENCES FOR THE BACK

Restorative yoga will bring your back to a comfortable state. There are a lot of exercises people do to strengthen the back, but to balance those active exercises, these passive postures are essential to your healing.

LOWER BACK PAIN

There are many culprits of lower back pain: Repetitive movements, bad posture, and weak stomach muscles all can lead to a variety of issues, including herniated discs and strained ligaments and muscles in the lower back. Even stress can play a role in back pain. When your body experiences stress and tension, the muscles in the back can tighten and strain in response. Emotional issues can also manifest as back pain. Fortunately, all of these culprits for lower back pain can be relieved with restorative yoga postures. With the postures in the following sequences, the muscles in the lower back are allowed to relax and the tension that is causing the pain is released. As you connect to your breath, let go of any emotions that arise as you hold the postures for the prescribed length of time.

TIME: 30 minutes

YOU NEED:
- Mat
- Wall
- Chair
- Bolster
- 2 blocks
- 2 blankets (Long Roll Fold)
- Sandbag (optional)
- Eye pillow (optional)

SHORT SEQUENCE

WHAT TO DO

1. Do three rounds of **Cat/Cow Tilts with Feet on Wall**. Be mindful of your breath as you inhale for the cow tilt and exhale for the cat tilt. This will relax your diaphragm, and help relax your back.

2. Sit for **Seated Twist (Option 2)**. Hold each side for at least three cycles of inhalation and exhalation.

3. Set up for **Supported Bound Angle Pose (either Option 1 or 2)**. Hold for fifteen minutes. Make sure your lower back comes right up to the bolster so that it is fully supported. If desired, drape a blanket over your legs.

4. Rest in **Savasana** for ten minutes. In addition to the regular pose instructions, it will be helpful here to put a sandbag on the lower abdomen to help relax the back. An eye pillow makes a nice addition here as well.

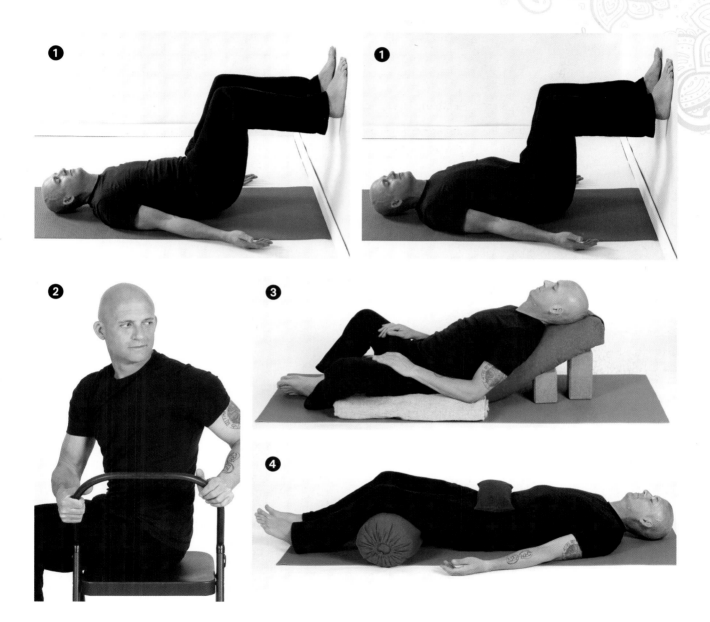

TIME: 75 minutes

YOU NEED:

- Mat
- Strap
- 2 blankets (Long Roll Fold, Square Fold, Head Rest Fold)
- Wall
- 2 blocks
- Bolster
- Chair
- Sandbag
- Eye pillow (optional)

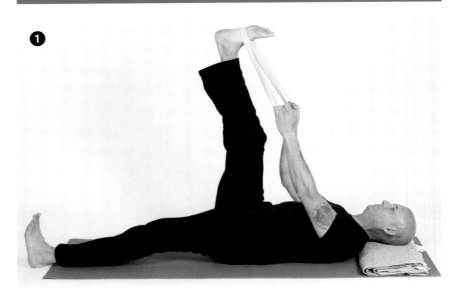

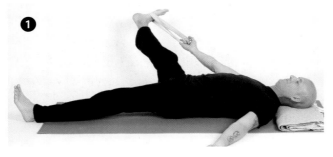

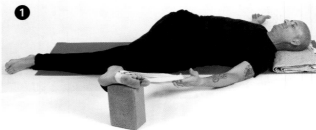

WHAT TO DO

1. Lie on your back for **Extended Hand to Foot Pose, Supine**. For this sequence, place a blanket under your head for neck support. While lying on your back, hold each leg up, out to the side, and across your body for one minute each before switching legs. Remember to use a strap folded in half under your foot as you move through the three leg positions to help with the stretch.

2. Move to the wall for **Wall Downward-Facing Dog**. Hold for four minutes.

3. From here, move into **Wall Half-Triangle Forward Bend**. Hold for four minutes, switching your legs after two minutes.

4. Lower to the floor for **Blanket Roll in 3 Positions**. Spend two minutes in each position.

5. Transition to **Simple Bridge with Block or Bolster under Hips**. For this sequence, use the block instead of the bolster. Hold for six minutes.

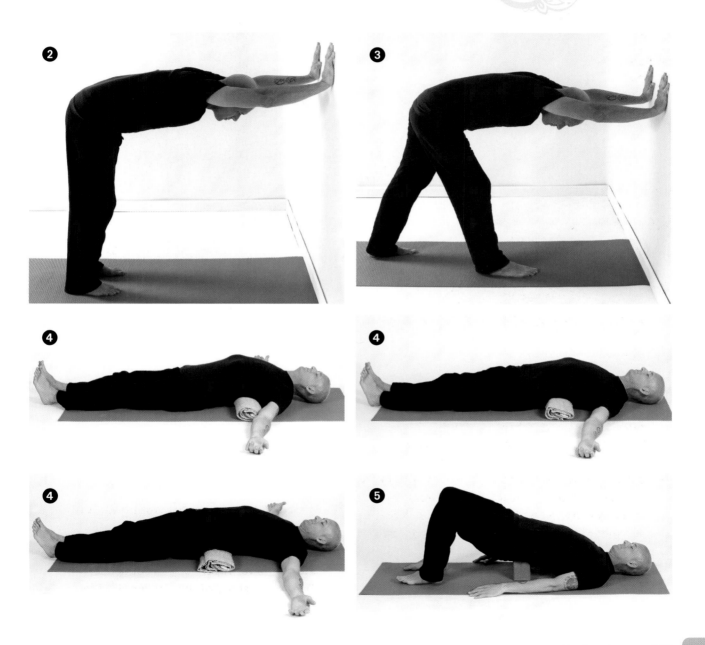

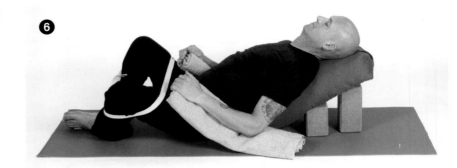

6. Remove the block and let your back rest on the floor. Gently knock your knees together to help the back relax. Once relaxed, move into **Supported Bound Angle Pose (Option 3)**. For this sequence, loop the strap around your knees instead of around your waist, as described in the variation sidebar for this pose option. Hold this pose for twelve minutes.

7. Come into **Child's Pose (Option 1)**. Hold for eight minutes.

8. Move into **Belly Down Twist over Bolster**. Hold for three minutes each side.

9. Move into **Legs on Chair**, and place a sandbag on your lower abdomen for the last fifteen minutes of your practice. This will act as your final relaxation pose.

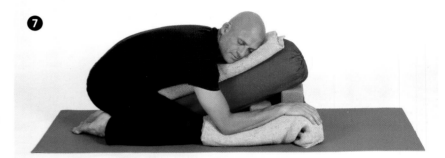

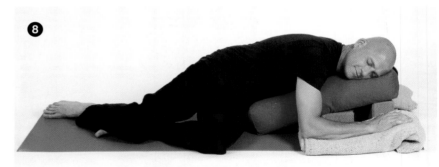

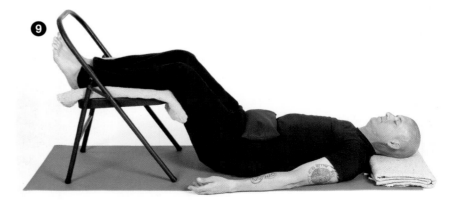

SCIATICA

TIME: 35 minutes

YOU NEED:
- Mat
- Wall
- Bolster
- Eye pillow (optional)

For some, sciatica is the major source of lower back pain. Sciatica is caused by irritation of, or pressure on, the sciatic nerve, a major nerve that originates in the lower back. The pain starts at the buttocks and runs down the leg. Many times a herniated spinal disc, or the piriformis muscle (the muscle deep in the hip used to turn the thigh out) presses against the sciatic nerve, triggering sciatica. Sciatica can be very painful, but the following restorative yoga sequences can help release the hip structure and help you manage the pain.

SHORT SEQUENCE

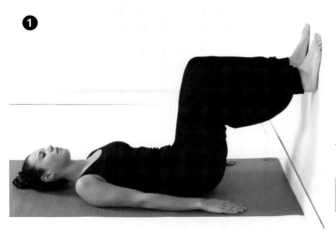

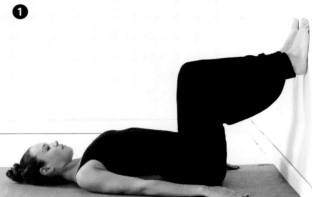

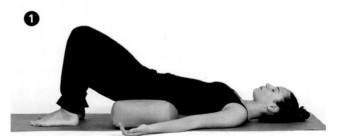

WHAT TO DO

1. Practice **Cat/Cow Tilts with Feet on Wall** for about four minutes, focusing on your breathing to relax the back.

2. Transition into **Simple Bridge with Block or Bolster under Hips**, using a bolster under the lower back. Try to relax down into the bolster. Hold this pose for six minutes.

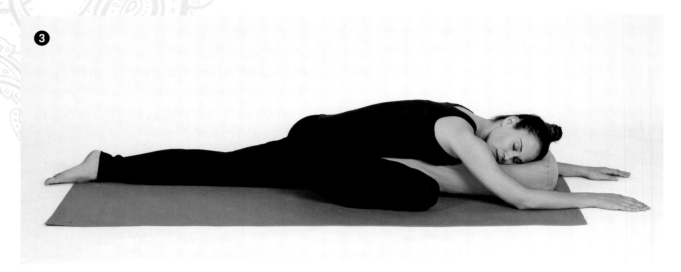

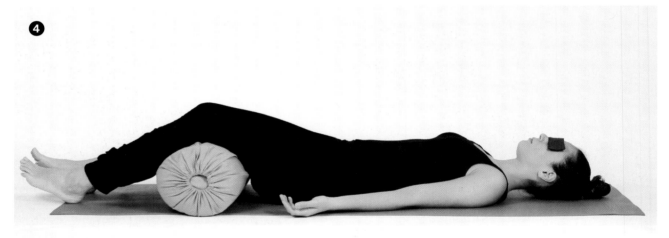

3. Transition into **Pigeon Pose with Bolster**. Hold for five minutes on each side.

4. Set up for **Savasana**. Place a bolster under your knees and hold the pose for fifteen minutes. Use an eye pillow for deeper relaxation.

TIME: 58 minutes

YOU NEED:

- Mat
- Wall
- Bolster
- 2 blocks
- 2 blankets (Rectangle Fold, Head Rest Fold, Square Fold)
- Eye pillow (optional)

WHAT TO DO

1. Practice **Cat/Cow Tilts with Feet on Wall** for about four minutes, focusing on your breathing to relax the back.

2. Move to the wall to practice **Wall Half-Triangle Forward Bend**, starting with your right foot forward, then switching to the left foot forward. Hold each foot for thirty seconds.

3. Make your way to the floor for **Child's Pose (Option 1)**. Raise yourself up higher using a second bolster on top of the first one, if this is too deep of a stretch. Hold the pose for ten minutes.

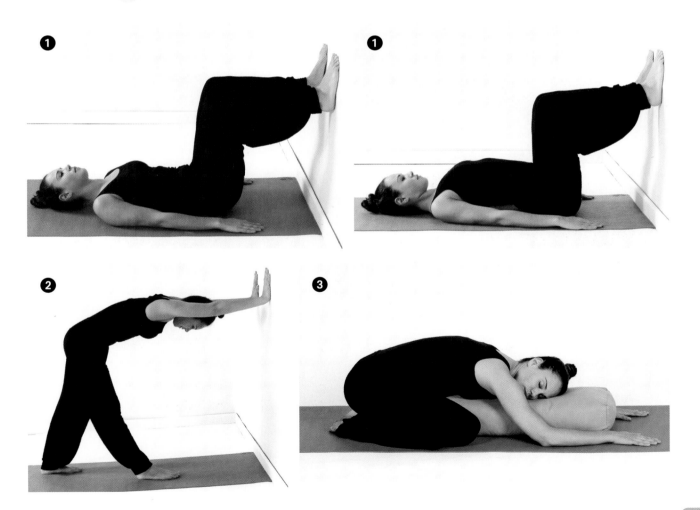

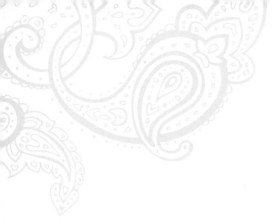

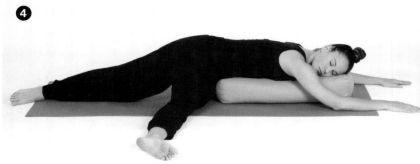

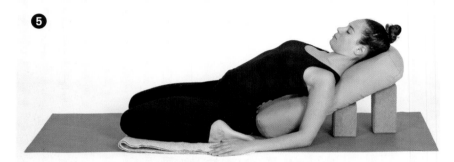

4. Move into **Scissored Legs Belly Down Twist**. Come to the right side first. Hold for three minutes on each side.

5. Move on to **Reclining Hero Pose (Option 2)**. This is a great pose to perform when you are experiencing sciatica, since it creates space in the hips and takes pressure off the nerve. Stay in this pose for twelve minutes.

6. Move into **Side Lying Stretch**. Hold for four minutes on each side.

7. Move into **Prone (on Belly) Savasana**. Hold for fifteen minutes.

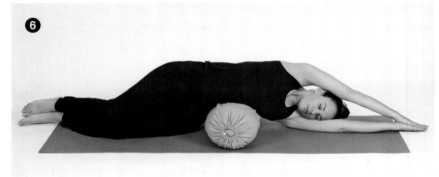

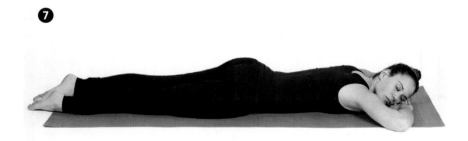

SEQUENCES FOR RESPIRATORY ISSUES

With restorative yoga, the poses are held long enough so that the beneficial effects of the practice have time to reach the major systems of the body—including the respiratory and immune systems. This is why restorative yoga can be especially beneficial for you when you are battling respiratory illnesses. Colds, flu, bronchitis, asthma, and other illnesses that restrict the chest with congestion and pain can be debilitating. When you are experiencing these symptoms, physical exercise can be an issue. Fortunately, restorative yoga is gentle enough to practice during this time, and can help with recovery.

GENERAL RESPIRATORY ILLNESSES

TIME: 30 minutes

YOU NEED:

- Mat
- Chair
- 2 blankets (Rectangle Fold and Square Fold)
- 2 bolsters
- Eye pillow (optional)

The poses in this sequence are designed to help you open your chest, reduce stress so that your immune system is allowed to work properly, and create a sense of relaxation to help you as you recover. Many of these poses and breathing techniques will also help your ability to breathe if your sinuses are congested.

SHORT SEQUENCE

WHAT TO DO

1. Sit in the chair. Center with **Alternate Nostril Breathing**. Practice for about four minutes. Be still for a few minutes afterward, to notice how your breathing is clearer.

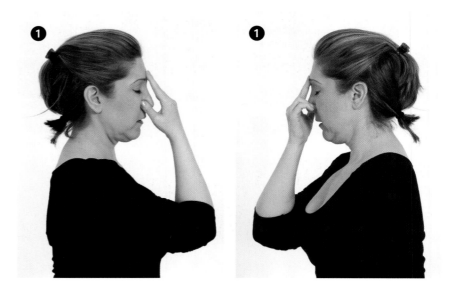

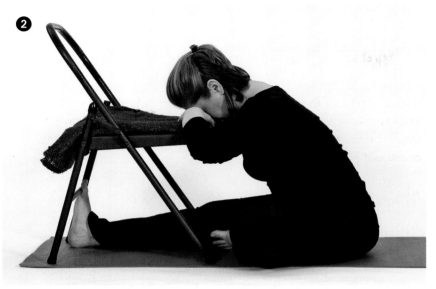

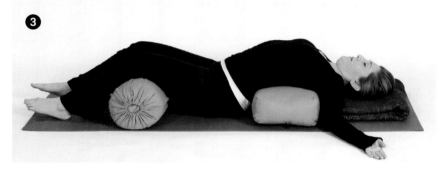

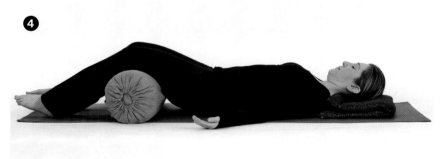

2. Move to **Chair Forward Bend (Option 2)**. Stretch three minutes for each leg.

3. Set up for **Heart Opening Pose**. Prop your head with a blanket if you need support, and place a blanket on you for added warmth, if needed. Hold the pose for ten minutes.

4. Come to **Savasana**. Hold for the remaining ten minutes of your practice.

TIME: 45 minutes

YOU NEED:
- Mat
- Chair
- 2 blankets (Square Fold and Rectangle Fold)
- 2 bolsters
- Eye pillow (optional)

WHAT TO DO

1. Sit in the chair. Center with **Alternate Nostril Breathing**. Practice for about four minutes. Be still for a few minutes afterward, to notice how your breathing is clearer.

2. Move to **Chair Forward Bend (Option 2)**. Stretch three minutes for each leg.

3. Move to the floor for **Revolved Abdomen Pose**. Feel the stretch deeply in your sides. Hold each side for three minutes each.

4. Transition to **Reclining Bridge Pose (Option 1)**. Use any props here to make yourself comfortable, such as a blanket under your head. Hold for ten minutes.

5. Come to **Legs on Chair** for your final relaxation. If desired, cover yourself with a blanket for warmth and use an eye pillow to really settle in. Take at least eight minutes here to allow yourself the full benefit of the pose.

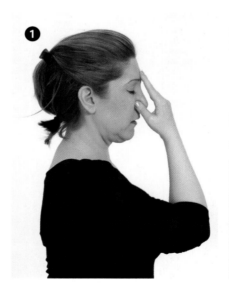
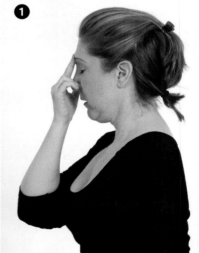

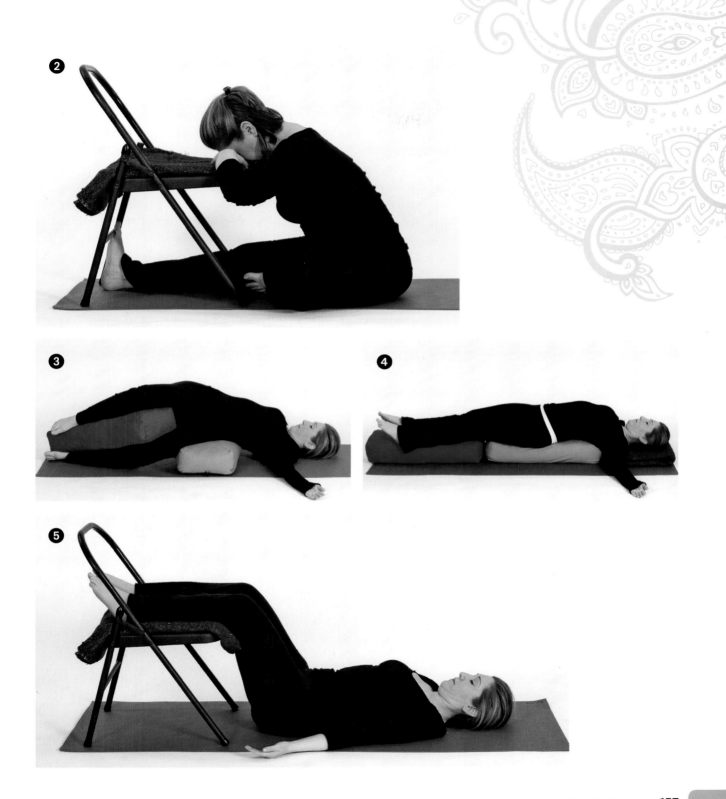

ASTHMA

Asthma sufferers can benefit greatly from restorative yoga. The practice of better postures that open the rib cage and build shoulder strength can help open the muscles that control breathing, helping asthmatics take in and breathe out air more fully. Naturally, breathing exercises in yoga can be especially beneficial to asthmatics as well. Building the power of your exhalation has been proven useful to helping asthmatics gain control over their breath. To that end, the following sequences focus on exercises that open the front body and help you develop control over your breath.

TIME: 30 minutes

YOU NEED:
- Mat
- 2 bolsters
- Blanket (Head Rest Fold or Rectangle Fold)
- Sandbag
- Eye pillow (optional)

SHORT SEQUENCE

WHAT TO DO

1. Begin by practicing **Breath with Pause**. Remember the pause comes after exhaling. Practice this for approximately four minutes.

2. Lie down on a mat to practice **Diaphragmatic Breath**. For this sequence, place a sandbag on your belly. Take full, deep breaths as you focus on feeling the breath in your belly, and the weight of the sandbag as your abdomen rises and falls. Practice this for three minutes.

3. Transition to **Cross Bolster Pose** and hold for about ten minutes.

4. Move into **Savasana**. You may keep a bolster underneath your knees and a sandbag on your chest, if desired. Hold for fifteen minutes.

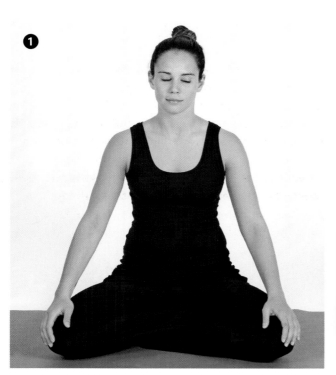

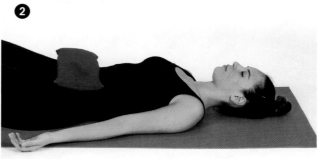

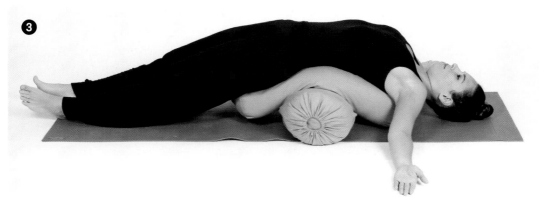

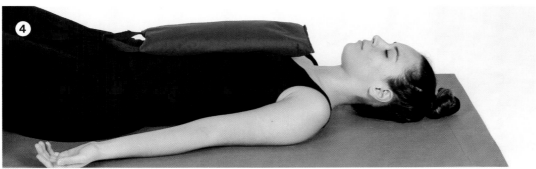

TIME: 75 minutes

YOU NEED:
- Mat
- Strap
- Bolster
- 2 blocks
- Blanket (Square Fold and Rectangle Fold)
- Sandbag
- Wall
- Eye pillow (optional)

WHAT TO DO

1. Begin by practicing **Breath with Pause**. Remember the pause comes after exhaling. Practice this for approximately four minutes.

2. Practice **Shoulder Stretches** for approximately two minutes.

3. Move into **Simple Bridge with Block or Bolster under Hips**. For this sequence, use a bolster and hold for fifteen minutes.

4. Transition to **Reclining Hero Pose (Option 1)**. If your feet cramp, make sure to raise your seat with a block so that it's comfortable for you to lie back. Hold this pose for ten minutes.

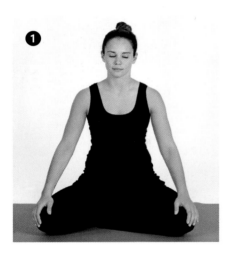

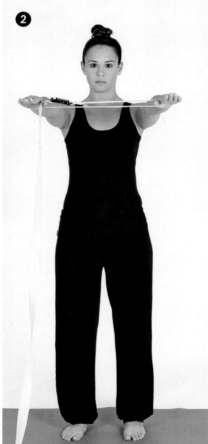

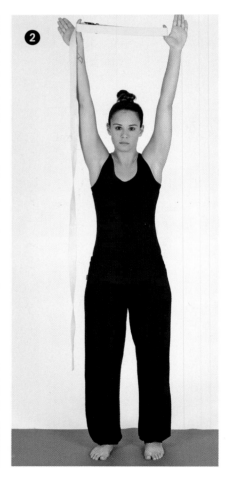

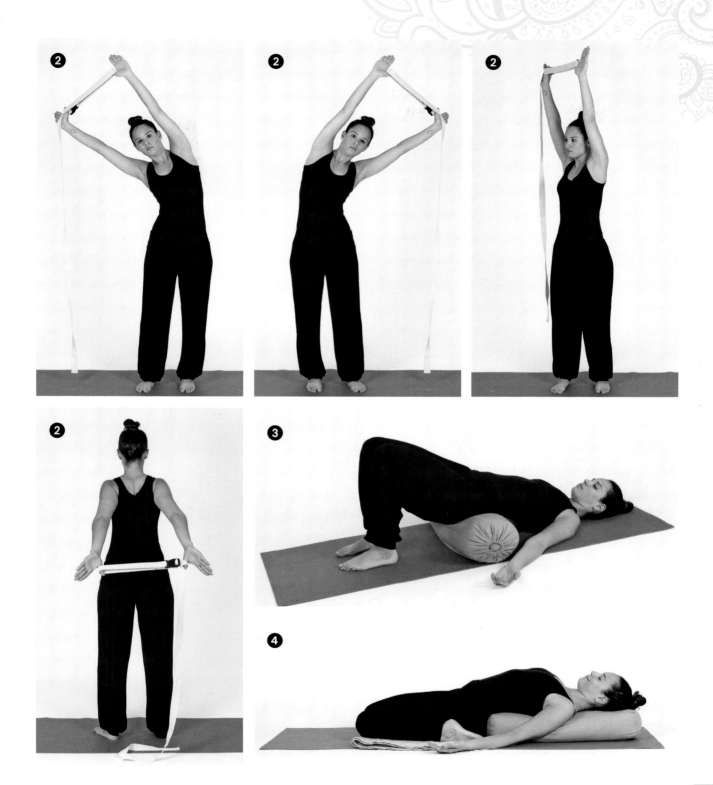

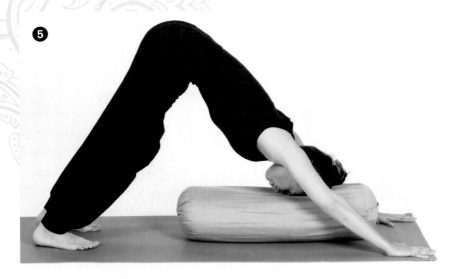

5. Move on to **Down Dog with Head on Block or Bolster**. Use the bolster for this sequence. Rest here for three minutes.

6. Come into **Legs Up the Wall Pose Without Bolster**. Place a sandbag on your lower abdomen. Hold this pose for twelve minutes.

7. Move the sandbag to your chest for **Savasana**. Hold the pose for fifteen minutes.

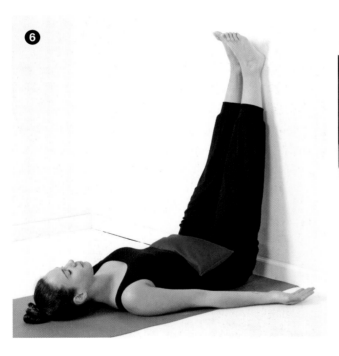

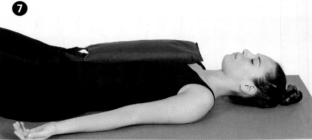

YOGIC WISDOM

Asthma can cause a lot of anxiety. The nervous system's automatic responses to an asthmatic attack can be debilitating. The effect of restorative yoga can help prevent or mitigate the anxiety-producing responses of the nervous system when they are triggered, thereby reducing the severity of asthma attacks when they occur.

SEQUENCES FOR MENTAL HEALTH

Restorative yoga encourages one to relax and to focus on the present moment, creating a more tranquil state of mind. Those who practice restorative yoga—and these sequences in particular—regularly will be able to create an overall sense of well-being in their lives. It has been shown that not only does the practice create calm, but also it creates a more positive sense of self by increasing serotonin production in the body, whereas low serotonin levels can cause depression.

DEPRESSION

More and more studies are showing that yoga can have a therapeutic effect on depression. Because yoga practice helps boost serotonin levels and decrease cortisol levels, it mimics the benefits of antidepressants. Restorative yoga in particular can be helpful for those suffering from depression. Holding the poses at length helps to create a better mind/body connection, which can help create an empowering sense of control over life situations. Back bends, which open up the heart chakra area, are usually very therapeutic for people who suffer from depression; they are featured in the following sequences. Some people with depression initially find it difficult to really relax in restorative poses. If you have trouble, try some active yoga postures first, then turn to restorative poses. Also, focus on extending the length of time that you exhale, which will help you relax.

TIME: 35 minutes

YOU NEED:
- Mat
- Wall
- 2 bolsters
- 2 blankets (Head Rest Fold and Rectangle Fold)
- Eye pillow (optional)

SHORT SEQUENCE

WHAT TO DO

1. Come to a comfortable seated position to practice **Breath with Pause**. Do this for a few minutes.

2. Move onto **Cat/Cow Tilts with Feet on Wall**. Practice for about two minutes.

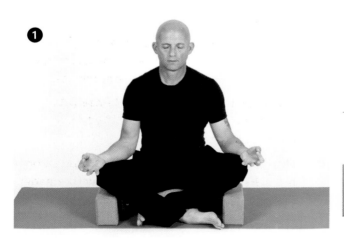

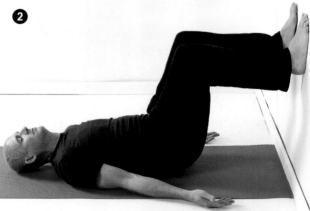

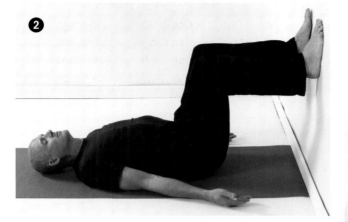

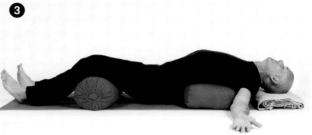

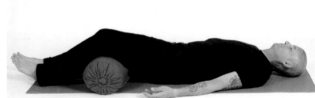

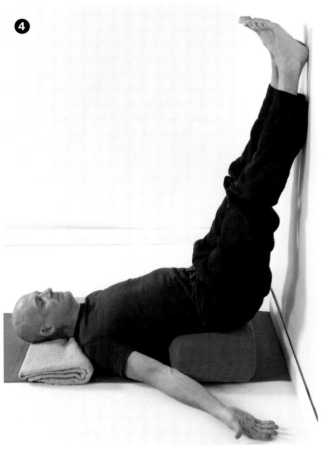

3. Set up for **Heart Opening Pose**, using one bolster under your knees and one under your upper back. Hold for about eight minutes.

4. Transition to **Legs Up the Wall Pose with Bolster** for about ten minutes. Try to fully relax in this pose.

5. Move onto **Savasana**. Hold for ten minutes or more. Feel free to use an eye pillow for deeper relaxation.

TIME: 1 hour

YOU NEED:

- Mat
- Wall
- 2 blocks
- 2 bolsters
- 2 blankets (Small Square Fold, Head Rest Fold, Rectangle Fold, Square Fold)
- Chair
- Eye pillow (optional)

WHAT TO DO

1. Seat yourself comfortably. Feel free to use a blanket in the Small Square Fold under your bottom for comfort, and/or sit against a wall for back support to practice **Breath with Pause**. Do this for a few minutes.

2. Move onto **Cat/Cow Tilts with Feet on Wall**. Practice for about two minutes.

3. Move onto **Simple Bridge with Block or Bolster under Hips**, using a block under your lower back. Hold this pose for six minutes. When you come out of the pose, lift your hips and remove the block, rest on your back for a minute, and roll to your right before you come up to a sitting position.

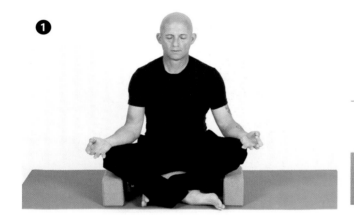

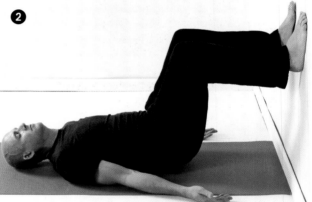

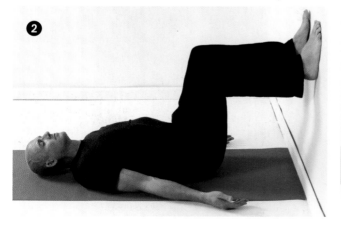

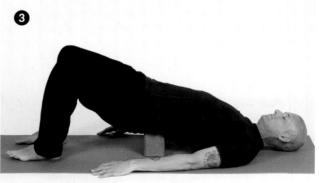

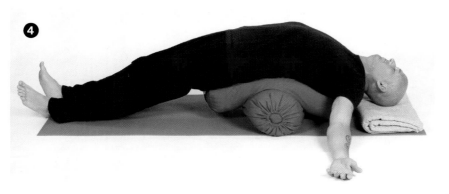

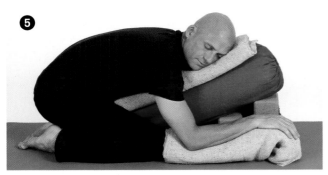

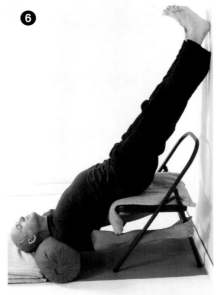

4. Next, set up for **Cross Bolster Pose**. Focus on taking full, complete breaths here. Stay in this pose for ten minutes.

5. Move into **Child's Pose (Option 1)** and hold for ten minutes.

6. Set up for **Chair Shoulder Stand** and hold the pose for ten minutes. When you transition out of this pose, remember to lower yourself down to the bolster and roll to your side.

7. Keep the bolster where it is and then place another bolster perpendicular to it along the center of the mat, creating a T-shape, and move into **Legs on Chair** for the final relaxation. Hold for fifteen minutes. Use an eye pillow for a deeper sense of relaxation, if desired.

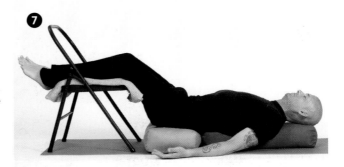

ANXIETY

TIME: 40 minutes

YOU NEED:
- Mat
- Bolster
- Chair
- Wall
- 2 blankets (Head Rest Fold, Square Fold, Rectangle Fold)
- 2 blocks
- Sandbag
- Eye pillow (optional)

Oftentimes long-term anxiety sufferers are prescribed medication to alleviate their anxiety symptoms, but restorative yoga can manage the symptoms in a less disruptive way to the body. The sequences in this section focus on poses that help relax the nervous system and the parts of the body that typically store increased tension from anxiety. These sequences, if done consistently over time, can be a powerful way to reprogram your body's automatic responses to stress, and reduce anxiety.

SHORT SEQUENCE

THREADS OF THOUGHT

Yama niyama-āsana prāṇ āyāma pratyāhāra dhāraṇā dhyāna samādhayo

Respect for others (yama) and yourself (niyama); harmony with: your body through postures (asana); your vital energy through breath control (pranayama); your thoughts through concentration (dharana); and your emotions through withdrawing from your senses (pratyahara); and finally, the practice of meditation (dhyana)—this is the path to enlightenment (samadhi).

WHAT TO DO

1. Bring yourself into **Savasana** on the floor. Practice **Apa Japa Breath** for five minutes to become aware of your breath.

2. Move into **Simple Bridge with Block or Bolster under Hips**, using a bolster. Hold this pose for five minutes.

3. Transition into **Belly Down Twist over Bolster**. Hold for three minutes on each side.

4. Set up for **Chair Forward Bend (Option 1)**. Cross legs for three minutes, and then change cross and hold for another three minutes.

5. Move to the wall for **Legs Up the Wall Pose with Bolster**. Hold the pose for ten minutes.

6. Finish with **Savasana**, placing a bolster under your knees and a sandbag on your belly. Hold the pose for ten minutes. If desired, use an eye pillow to deepen relaxation.

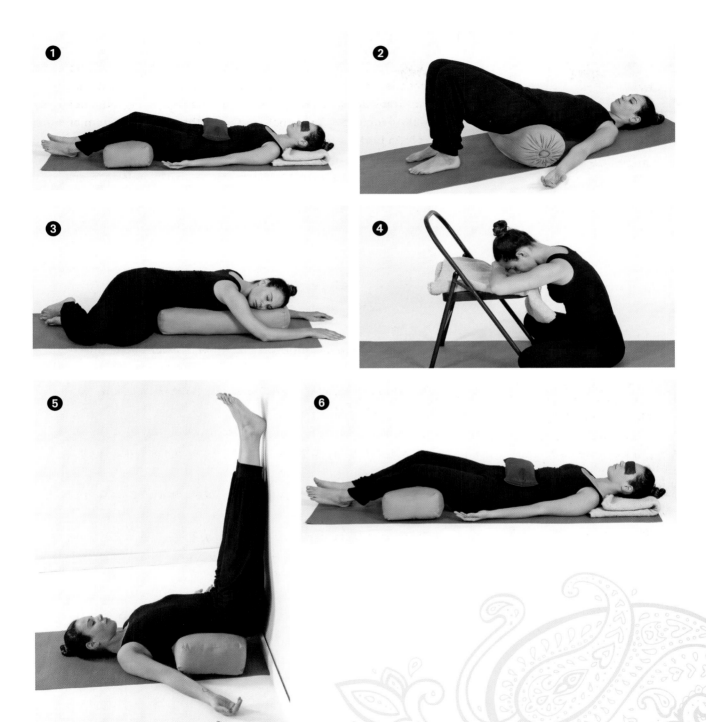

TIME: 75 minutes

YOU NEED:
- Mat
- 2 blocks
- Wall
- 2 blankets (Rectangle Fold, Head Rest Fold, Half Fold)
- 2 bolsters
- Sandbag
- Eye pillow (optional)

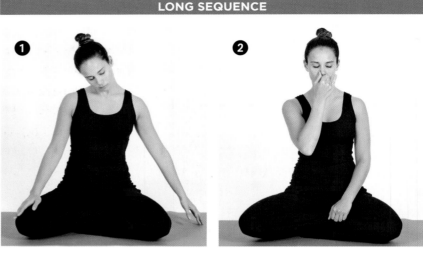

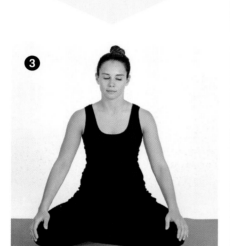

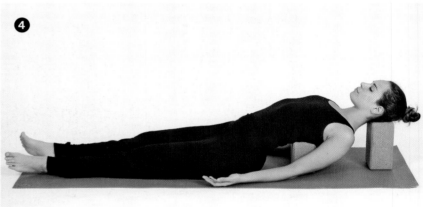

WHAT TO DO

1. Begin by practicing **Neck Stretches**. Hold the stretch on each side for at least a couple of breaths, and lengthen it if you can by stretching your arms toward the floor—you want to really feel a full release in your neck area.

2. Move to a comfortable seated position on the floor and practice ten complete rounds of **Alternate Nostril Breathing**. When you are done, breathe normally for a minute or two.

3. Next, practice **Ujjaii Breath (Option 1)** for about two minutes, increasing the length of the exhalation with each breath.

4. Transition into **Fish Pose with Blocks or Bolster**, using blocks. Hold the pose for five minutes.

5. Move to the wall for **Legs Up the Wall Pose with Bolster**. Use an eye pillow to deepen your sense of relaxation. Hold the pose for ten minutes.

6. Set up for **Child's Pose (Option 1)**, placing a sandbag on your back. Hold for ten minutes.

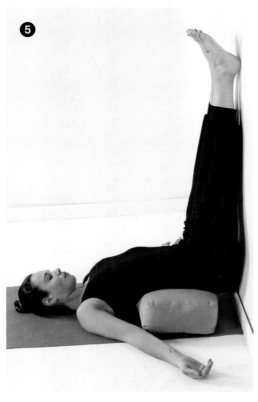

7. Practice **Pigeon Pose with Bolster** for five minutes on each side.

8. Keep your bolster and shift into **Revolved Abdomen Pose**, holding it for three minutes on each side.

9. Come into **Supported Bound Angle Pose (Option 4)**. Use an eye pillow for a deeper sense of relaxation. Swaddle yourself. Stay in this pose for twelve minutes or longer.

10. Move into **Prone (on Belly) Savasana**. Hold for twelve minutes.

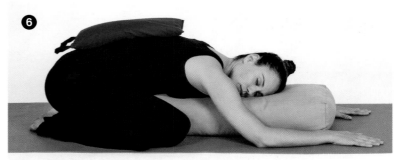

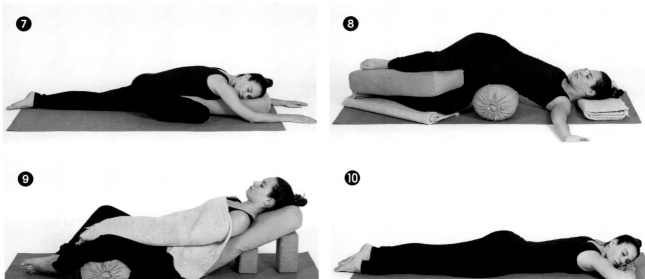

STRESS

We need to relax. Our society is almost *always* on the go. We work more and more, and take less and less downtime. If this sounds like you, then you need to find some time to relax. If you are regularly stressed, then your body eventually can't keep up. Your cortisol levels (the stress hormone) are constantly raised, which leads to adrenal burnout, and when the adrenals burn out it sets off a chain reaction that unbalances your hormones, circulatory system, and neural function. Fortunately, restorative yoga is the key to optimal health: It can be incorporated into even the busiest schedule, and creates a relaxation response that resets the nervous system. The following sequences focus on releasing tension by bringing more breath into the body, and making you feel more grounded.

TIME: 40 minutes

YOU NEED:
- Mat
- Bolster
- Wall
- 2 blankets (Head Rest Fold and Rectangle Fold)
- 2 blocks (optional)
- Eye pillow (optional)

SHORT SEQUENCE

WHAT TO DO

1. Lie down or sit comfortably to practice **Diaphragmatic Breath**. Stay here for about three minutes.

2. Come up for **Down Dog with Head on Block or Bolster**. For this sequence, place a bolster under your head and hold for three minutes.

3. Move onto your knees for **Child's Pose (Option 1)**, with your head turned to each side for five minutes.

4. Move into the **Legs Up the Wall Pose with Bolster** for ten minutes. As you hold the pose, feel the tension draining from you, and the support of the floor under your back.

5. Move into **Savasana**. If desired, place an eye pillow on your eyes for an additional relaxing effect. Hold the pose for ten minutes.

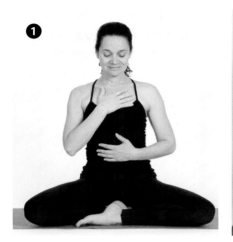

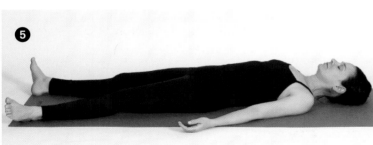

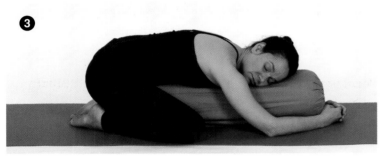

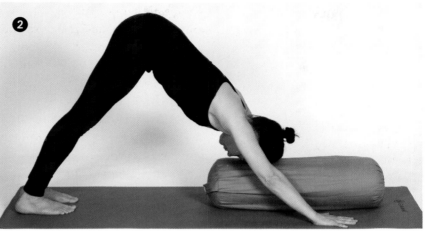

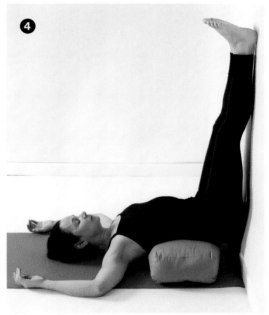

TIME: 1 hour

YOU NEED:

- Mat
- Strap
- 2 blankets (Head Rest Fold and Rectangle Fold)
- 2 blocks
- 2 bolsters
- Sandbag
- Wall
- Eye pillow (optional)

WHAT TO DO

1. Lie down or sit comfortably to practice **Diaphragmatic Breath** and begin to relax. Stay here for about three minutes.

2. Transition into **Extended Hand to Foot Pose, Supine**. Hold one leg straight up, then out to the side, then across your body for one minute each. Switch to the other leg and repeat.

3. Move into **Belly Down with Bolster at Hip**. Rest your forehead on your hands, and hold for five minutes.

4. Shift into **Child's Pose (Option 1)** and place a sandbag on your back. Hold for ten minutes. Your forehead can be centered down, or you may turn your head to rest your cheek on your hands for five minutes, then turn your head the other way and rest for the last five minutes. Be aware of the weight of the sandbag on your back.

5. Move into **Supported Bound Angle Pose (Option 4)**. Hold the pose for ten minutes.

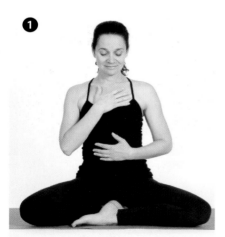

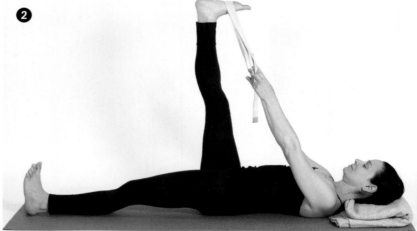

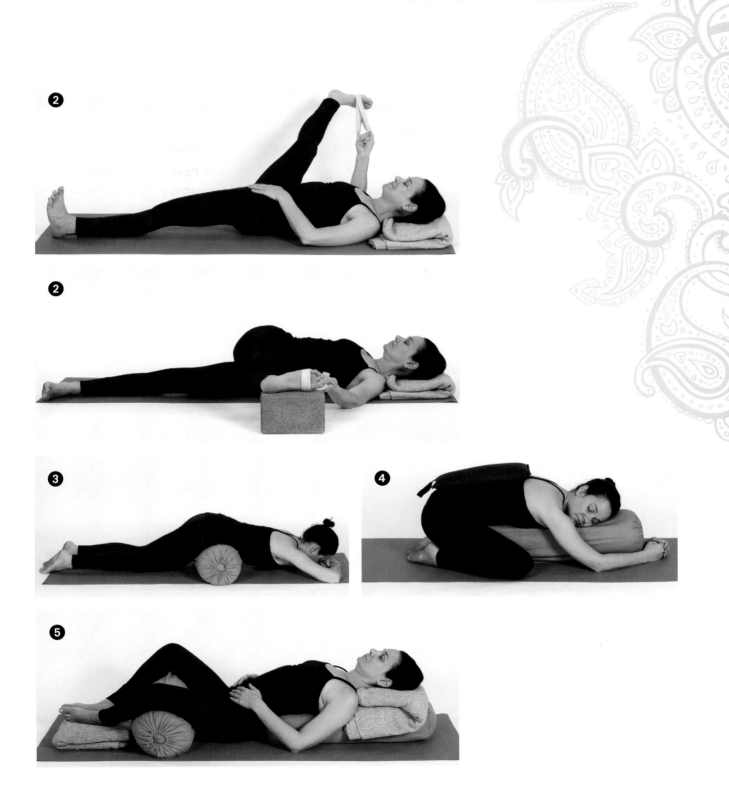

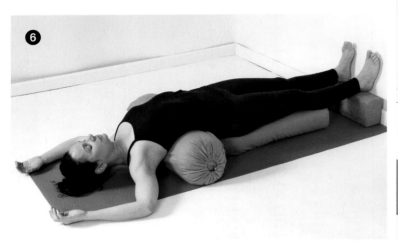

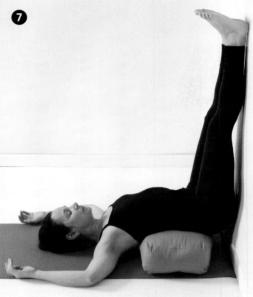

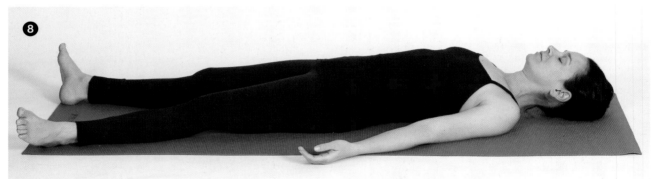

6. Move into **Reclining Bridge Pose (Option 2)** and focus on opening your chest. Hold the pose for ten minutes.

7. Transition into **Legs Up the Wall Pose with Bolster**. Feel the tension draining from you, and the support of the floor under your back. Hold this pose for ten minutes.

8. Finish by moving into **Savasana**. Use an eye pillow here to deepen your sense of relaxation. Hold the pose for ten minutes.

SEQUENCES FOR DIGESTIVE DISORDERS

Posture is in an important factor that can be overlooked in people suffering from intestinal issues. When we focus on correcting specific habitual postures that compress the intestines, particularly positions where the head is tilted forward, we begin to help the body regain normal bowel functions. Twists are especially helpful in stimulating the muscles in the abdomen that play a role in digestion. Stress can also be a factor in people dealing with intestinal problems. Stress clouds the mind, and when you become more aware of the body, you can better tune in to what the body is saying and reacting to. The postures in these sequences help to reduce stress and support the muscles in the abdomen to promote digestion.

COLITIS, CROHN'S, AND IRRITABLE BOWEL SYNDROME

TIME: 35 minutes

YOU NEED:
- Mat
- 2 bolsters
- 2 blankets (Open Fold, Square Fold, Rectangle Fold)
- 2 blocks
- Wall
- Chair
- Eye pillow (optional)

Stress is a major cause of inflammation, and when you have the diseases discussed in this section you want to decrease the inflammation as much as possible. Restorative yoga not only helps with stress levels, but the gentle stretches are very helpful in easing the stress-related tightness you may experience.

SHORT SEQUENCE

WHAT TO DO

1. Lie down to practice **Apa Japa Breath**. Focus on your thoughts. Every time a thought comes to your mind, tag it with a number, and let it go. You may find you may not even get to number ten. Do this for three minutes.

2. Move into **Supported Bound Angle Pose (Option 2)**. An extra blanket is a great addition here if needed. If you place it over your body, it provides a sense of relaxation with the added weight. Stay for about ten minutes.

3. Transition to **Chair Shoulder Stand** and hold for ten minutes. To come down from this pose, slide down to rest your lower back on the bolster and your legs on the chair for one minute.

4. Transition to **Legs on Chair** for final relaxation. For this sequence, use two bolsters in a T-shape and rest your legs on the chair. If you like, you can place a blanket over yourself and an eye pillow on your eyes. Hold this pose for about twelve minutes.

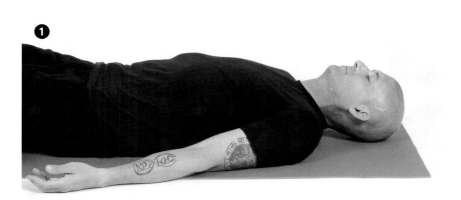

❶

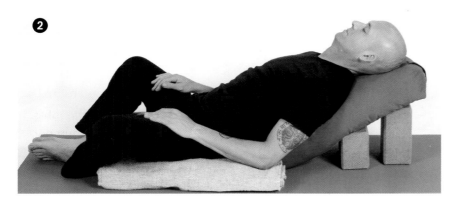

❷

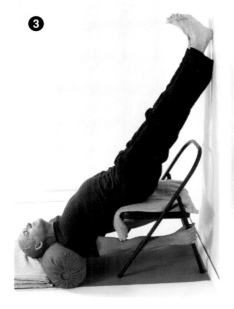

❸

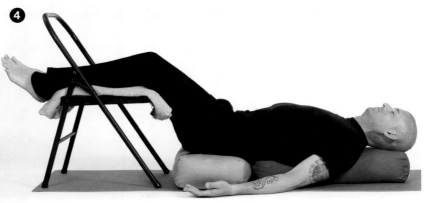

❹

TIME: 75 minutes

YOU NEED:
- Mat
- Strap
- 2 bolsters
- 2 blankets (Rectangle Fold, Square Fold, Open Fold)
- 2 blocks
- Chair
- Wall
- Eye pillow (optional)

WHAT TO DO

1. Come to a comfortable seated position on the floor or chair with a straight spine. Begin by breathing as you practice the **Straw** visualization. Do this for five minutes.

2. Lie back for **Wind Relieving Pose**. Practice three times on each side. A blanket under your head here can be good.

3. Take your strap and move to **Extended Hand to Foot Pose, Supine**. While lying on your back, hold each leg up, out to the side, and across your body for one minute each before switching legs.

4. Move into **Supported Bound Angle Pose (Option 2)**. An extra blanket is a great addition here if desired. Stay here for at least ten minutes.

5. Then move to **Belly Down with Bolster at Hip**. For this sequence, however, place the bolster at your belly, not at your hips. Stay in this pose for eight minutes.

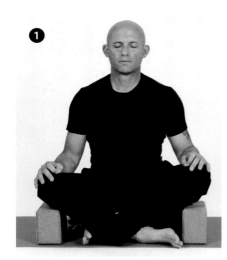

1

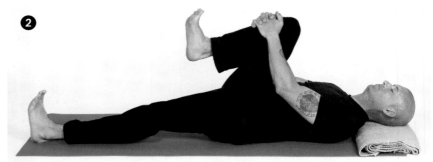

2

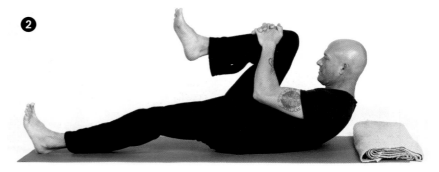

2

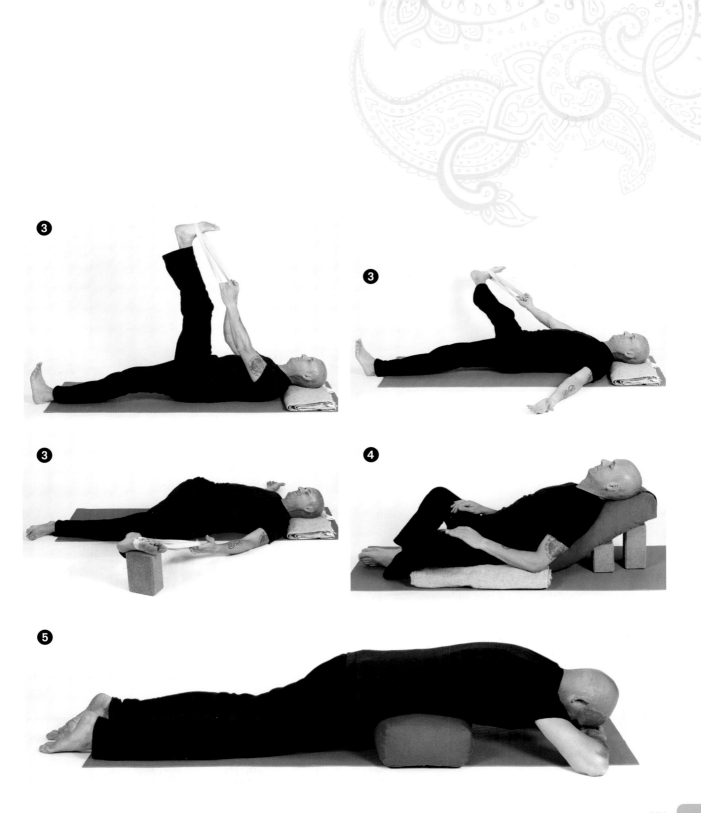

❻

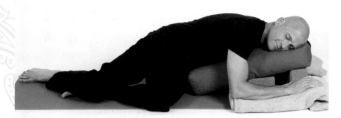

❼

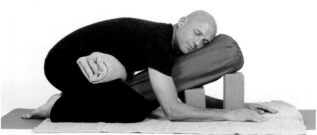

❽

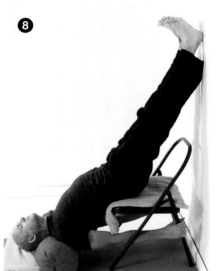

❾

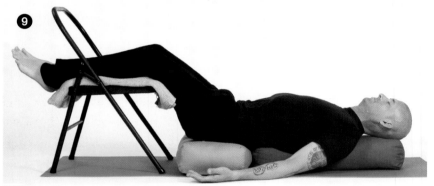

6. Transition to **Belly Down Twist over Bolster**. If desired, place a Rectangle Fold blanket at your lower abdomen. Stay on each side for four minutes.

7. Move into **Child's Pose (Option 1)**. Use the Rectangle Fold blanket at your lower abdomen before you fold forward. If desired, keep a blanket under your forehead to help make room for your nose so you can lower your head and breathe comfortably. Stay in this pose for ten minutes.

8. Set up for **Chair Shoulder Stand**. Stay here for three minutes.

9. Move into **Legs on Chair** for final relaxation. For this sequence, position the bolster in a T-shape for under your back and hips, and bring your legs to rest up on the chair. Hold this pose for fifteen minutes, if possible. An eye pillow is a wonderful addition for deeper relaxation, if desired.

> **YOGIC WISDOM**
>
> *If you are experiencing diarrhea, avoid twists.*

CONSTIPATION

In Ayurvedic thought, bowel function is ruled by the *apana*, or downward movement, in the body. It is especially an issue for those who have a Vata (air)-dominant doshic makeup, which is very common in our fast-paced society. People with this doshic makeup tend to have mucous membranes in the colon that are especially dry, which can cause constipation. The following restorative yoga sequences help to stimulate the muscles involved in elimination, and also work to make you feel more grounded to correct this Vata imbalance.

TIME: 40 minutes

YOU NEED:

- Mat
- Chair
- 2 blankets (Long Roll Fold, Rectangle Fold, Open Fold)
- 2 bolsters
- 2 blocks
- Wall
- Strap
- Eye pillow (optional)

SHORT SEQUENCE

WHAT TO DO

1. Begin in **Savasana** with a Long Roll Fold blanket under your knees. Stay here for three minutes.

2. Remain on your back and practice **Wind Relieving Pose** for three rounds on each leg.

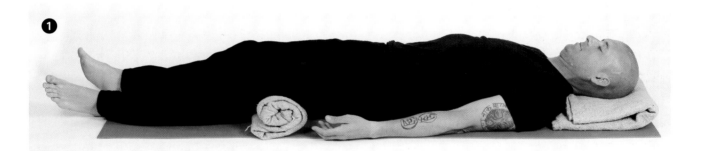

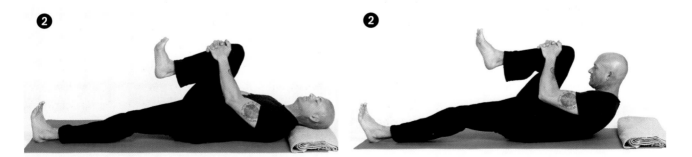

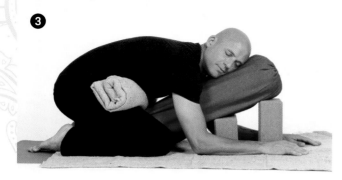

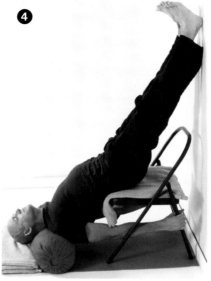

3. Move into **Child's Pose (Option 1)**. Use the Rectangle Fold blanket at your lower abdomen before you fold forward. Hold the pose for eight minutes.

4. Set up for **Chair Shoulder Stand** and stay in the pose for five minutes. As you lower down to come out of the pose, stay for two minutes with your lower back on the bolster and your tailbone dropping toward the floor.

5. Set up for **Revolved Abdomen Pose**, starting on your left side first. Stay there for two minutes before switching to your right side and repeating the pose for another two minutes.

6. Take your strap and transition into **Supported Bound Angle Pose (Option 3)** to support your legs. Hold for eight minutes.

7. Move into **Side Lying Savasana** on your left side. For this particular sequence, feel free to use an Open Fold blanket if you'd like. Hold for ten minutes or more.

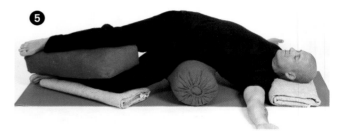

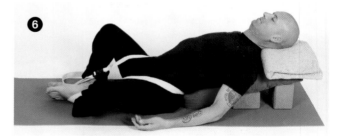

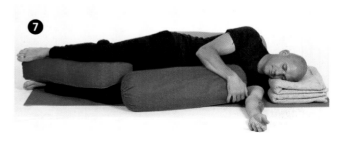

TIME: 1 hour

YOU NEED:
- Mat
- Chair
- 2 blankets (Rectangle Fold and Square Fold)
- 2 bolsters
- 2 blocks
- Wall
- Strap
- Eye pillow (optional)

WHAT TO DO

1. Practice **Wind Relieving Pose** for three rounds on each leg.

2. Come up to sit for a **Seated Twist (Option 2)**. Do three rounds per side.

3. Now that you are warmed up, move into **Child's Pose (Option 1)**. Use the Rectangle Fold blanket at your lower abdomen before you fold forward. Hold for ten minutes.

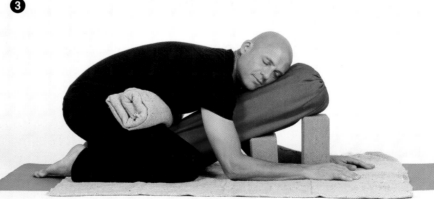

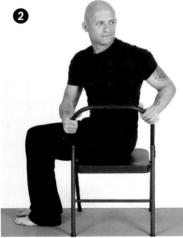

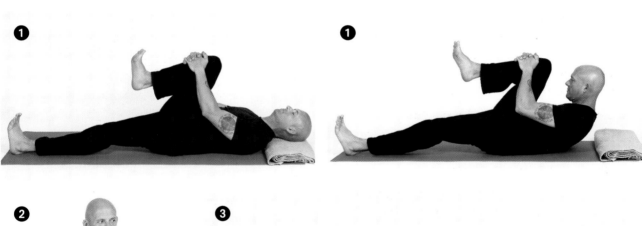

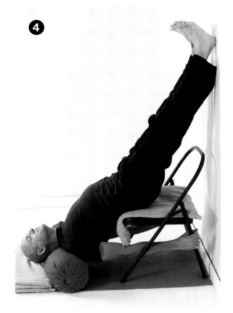

4. Next, move into **Chair Shoulder Stand**. Try to stay in this pose for ten minutes. As you lower down to come out of the pose, stay for three minutes with your lower back on the bolster and your tailbone dropping toward the floor.

5. Come into **Supported Bound Angle Pose (Option 3)**. Try to hold this pose for a minimum of ten minutes.

6. Move into **Scissored Legs Belly Down Twist** and hold for three minutes on each side. Start with your left hip to the bolster first.

7. Move into **Savasana** and hold the pose for fifteen minutes or longer. For this sequence, you will need to place a bolster under your knees and strap your legs above the knee. If desired, use an eye pillow for relaxation.

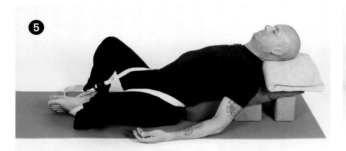

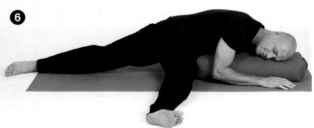

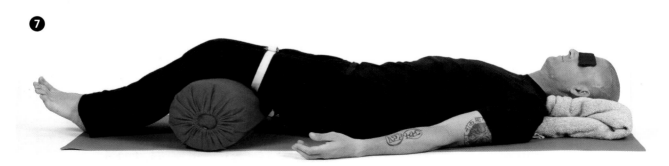

SEQUENCES FOR NEUROLOGICAL DISORDERS

Diseases that attack the nervous system affect not only your motor skills, but also brain function. By doing the restorative yoga sequences found in this section, you can positively affect the neurons that control the muscles as well as the brain. Relaxation techniques and mindful meditation also help with these disorders.

STROKE/HIGH BLOOD PRESSURE

TIME: 30 minutes

YOU NEED:
- Mat
- 2 blankets (Head Rest Fold and Rectangle Fold)
- 2 bolsters
- 2 blocks
- Strap
- Headwrap

Restorative yoga has been shown to lower blood pressure, which is one of the causes of strokes. Yoga also reduces the tendency of platelets to become clots. Once someone has experienced a stroke, restorative yoga can help bring him or her back to lead a normal life. Yoga has been shown to help recreate synapses in the brain that may have been lost or damaged, and therefore can help people rediscover movements or train the brain in new ways.

SHORT SEQUENCE

WHAT TO DO

1. Sit in a comfortable position with a straight spine. Begin by practicing the **Straw** visualization for four minutes. Then practice **Ujjaii Breath (Option 2)**. Focus on extending your exhalation. Do this for two minutes.

2. Take your strap and move to **Extended Hand to Foot Pose, Supine**. While lying on your back, hold each leg up, out to the side, and across your body for one minute each before switching legs.

3. Move into **Seated Twist (Option 1)**. Take three full breath cycles on each side.

4. Set up for **Supported Bound Angle Pose (Option 5)**. Hold this pose for eight minutes.

5. Move to **Savasana** with your head wrapped for ten minutes. To wrap your head, start with one end of the headwrap held against the side of your head, and begin to wrap it around your head on an angle from the lowest point to the highest point, making sure to cover the eyes and the forehead well. Attach the end of the wrap with the fasteners. Be sure to support your head properly with a Head Rest Fold blanket.

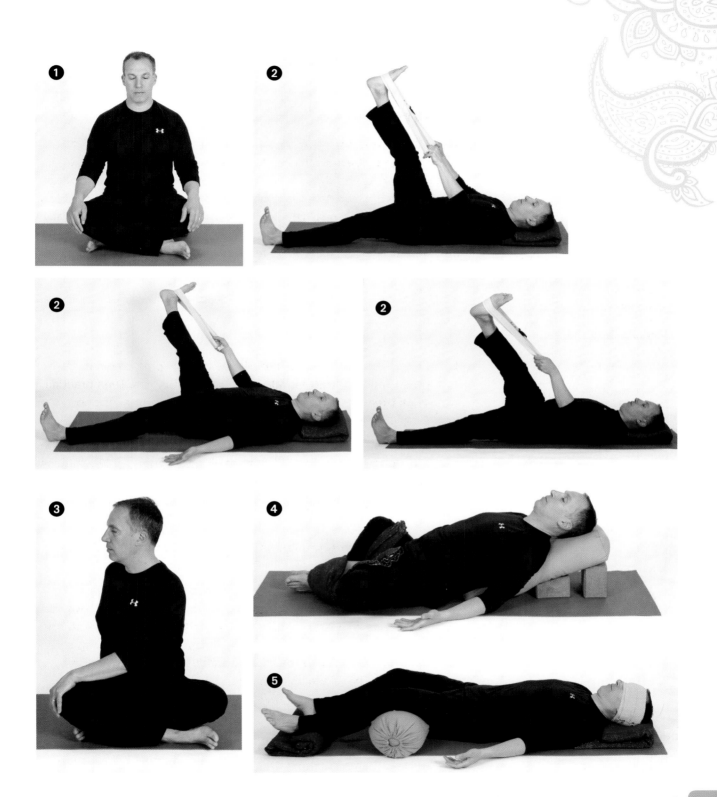

TIME: 1 hour

YOU NEED:

- Mat
- 2 blankets (Head Rest Fold and Rectangle Fold)
- 2 bolsters
- 2 blocks
- Strap
- Wall
- Headwrap

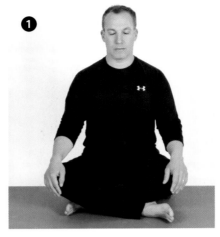

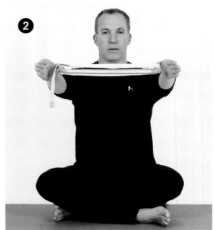

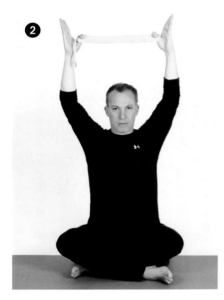

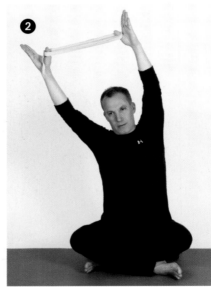

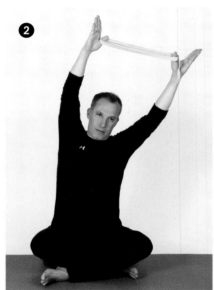

WHAT TO DO

1. Practice **Ujjaii Breath (Option 2)**. Focus on extending your exhalation.

2. Stay seated and do the **Shoulder Stretches**, repeating each variation three times.

3. Set up for **Fish Pose with Blocks or Bolster**. For this sequence, use a pair of blocks set up at either short and medium height, or medium and tall height. Hold for six minutes. Focus on inhaling and exhaling fully.

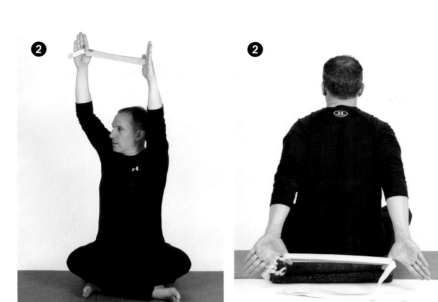

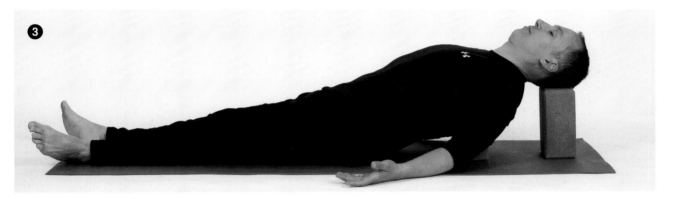

4. Roll to your right side for a few moments to adjust, then set up your bolster on an angle, using the blocks to support it, for **Fan Pose**. Sitting in **Fan Pose**, rest your torso on the bolster in front of you. You may need to use an additional bolster or blanket if you can't reach the bolster easily. Stay in this pose for eight minutes.

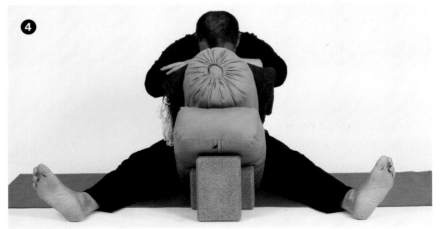

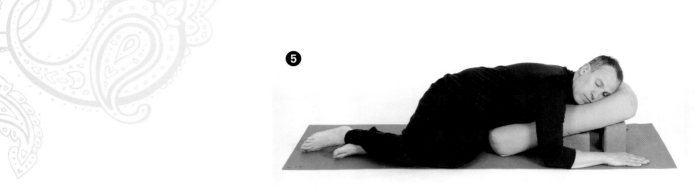

⑤

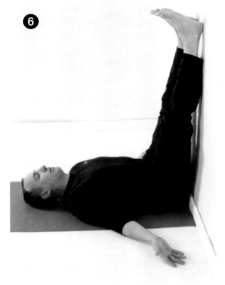

⑥

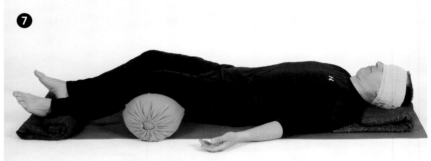

⑦

5. Move into **Belly Down Twist over Bolster**. Do this twist for three minutes on each side.

6. Bring yourself to the wall for **Legs Up the Wall Pose Without Bolster**. Hold the pose for ten minutes.

7. Move to **Savasana** with headwrap for fifteen minutes. To wrap your head, start with one end of the headwrap held against the side of your head, and begin to wrap it around your head on an angle from the lowest point to the highest point, making sure to cover the eyes and the forehead well. Attach the end of the wrap with the fasteners. Be sure to support your head properly with a Head Rest Fold blanket.

YOGIC WISDOM

If you are in any way uncomfortable in a pose, do not stay in the position. The agitation may raise your blood pressure. Make sure you are comfortable at all times, and feel free to use additional props as needed.

ALZHEIMER'S AND DEMENTIA

More and more research is starting to show that yoga and meditation are helpful to people dealing with dementia and Alzheimer's. Stress management and regular exercise are helpful in preventing and slowing down the progression of Alzheimer's and dementia, and restorative yoga can provide these things. During sleep, our brains clear away toxins. Since restorative yoga produces many of the chemical benefits of sleep, the following sequences can also help sufferers in this way.

TIME: 30 minutes

YOU NEED:

- Mat
- Wall
- Chair
- Bolster
- 2 blankets (Square Fold and Rectangle Fold)
- Eye pillow (optional)

SHORT SEQUENCE

WHAT TO DO

1. Seat yourself comfortably on the floor to practice **Apa Japa Breath**. Practice this for two minutes.

2. Move to the wall for **Wall Downward-Facing Dog**. Stay in the pose for two minutes.

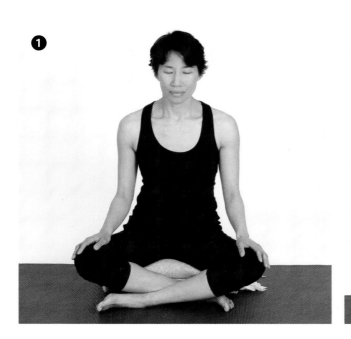

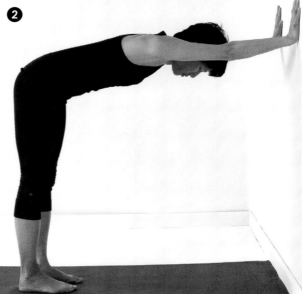

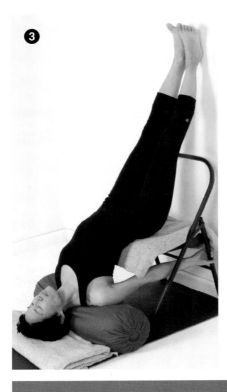

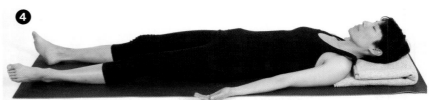

3. Set up for **Chair Shoulder Stand** and stay in the pose for six minutes. When your six minutes are up, slide down so your lower back is on the bolster and your legs are resting on the chair. Stay in this pose for eight minutes.

4. Lie down in **Savasana**. Hold for ten minutes. Use the eye pillow, if you desire.

WHAT TO DO

1. Begin by practicing **Ujjaii Breath (Option 1)** to bring heat into the body. Practice this for two minutes.

TIME: 1 hour

YOU NEED:
- Mat
- Chair
- 2 bolsters
- 2 blankets (Square Fold and Rectangle Fold)
- Wall
- Eye pillow (optional)

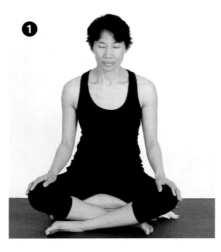

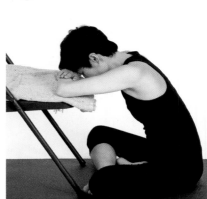

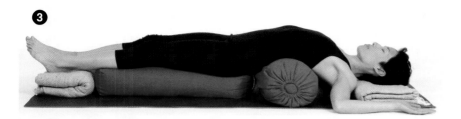

2. Move to your chair for **Chair Forward Bend (Option 1)**. Cross your legs for four minutes with the right leg in front, and four minutes with the left leg in front.

3. Set up for **Reclining Bridge Pose (Option 1)**, using the top bolster horizontally. Stay in this pose for ten minutes.

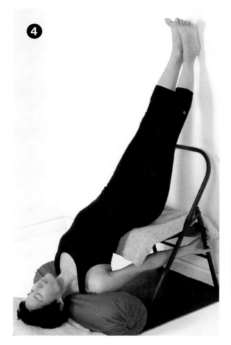

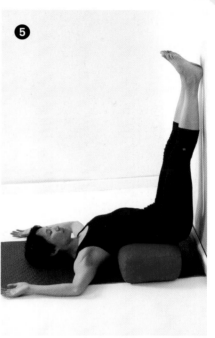

4. Move back to the chair for **Chair Shoulder Stand**. Stay in this pose for six minutes. Then slide down from the chair to rest your lower back on the bolster and your legs on the chair. Hold this pose for eight minutes.

5. Transition to the wall for **Legs Up the Wall Pose with Bolster**. Hold the pose for ten minutes.

6. Finish up in **Savasana**. Hold the pose for twelve minutes. Use the eye pillow, if desired.

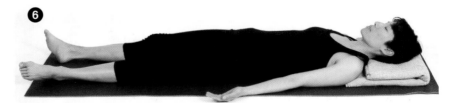

PARKINSON'S DISEASE

No two people with Parkinson's experience the disease the same way. However, restorative yoga can help make most of the symptoms a lot more bearable, no matter how the disease is experienced. Restorative yoga increases flexibility and range of motion, enhances posture, improves circulation, and helps people with Parkinson's feel more positive and less fatigued. The following sequences feature diaphragmatic breathing exercises, so pay special attention to your breathing as you practice all of the poses.

TIME: 40 minutes

YOU NEED:
- Mat
- 2 chairs
- Bolster
- 2 blocks
- 2 blankets (Rectangle Fold, Long Roll Fold, Head Rest Fold)
- Eye pillow (optional)

SHORT SEQUENCE

WHAT TO DO

1. Lie down or come to a comfortable seated position and practice **Diaphragmatic Breath** for three minutes.

2. Move into **Seated Twist (Option 1)**. Continue to deeply inhale and exhale for three cycles on each side.

3. Set up for **Child's Pose (Option 2)**. Stay in this pose for ten minutes.

4. Move to the floor for **Blanket Roll in 3 Positions**. Hold each position for two minutes each.

5. Set up for **Fish Pose with Blocks or Bolster**, using blocks for this particular sequence. Hold the pose for one minute.

6. Roll to your side and move the blocks away to set up for **Savasana**. Hold the pose for twelve minutes. Use the eye pillow, if you desire.

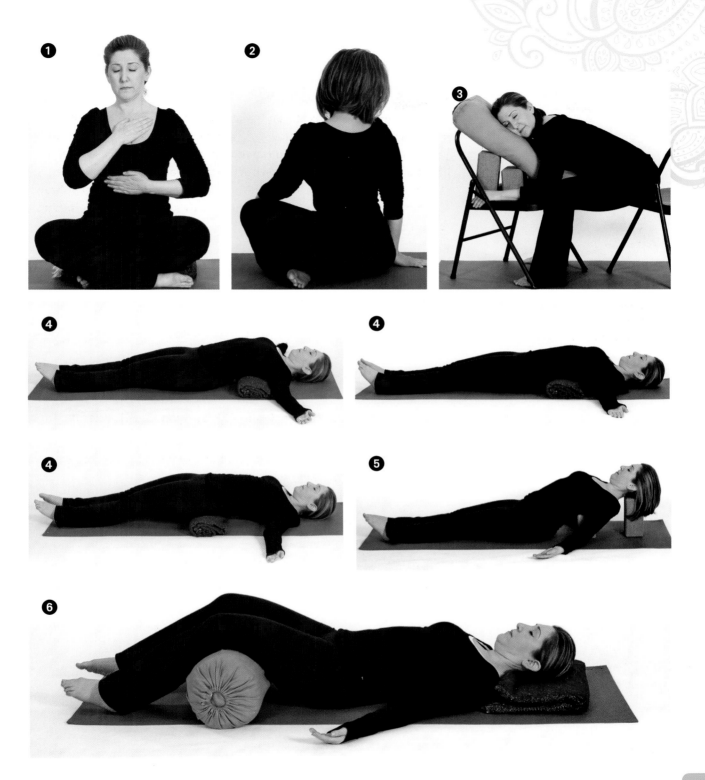

TIME: 1 hour

YOU NEED:

- Mat
- Chair
- 2 bolsters
- 2 blocks
- 2 blankets (Rectangle Fold and Square Fold)
- Eye pillow (optional)

WHAT TO DO

1. Lie down or come to a comfortable seated position and practice **Diaphragmatic Breath** for five minutes.

2. Practice **Revolved Abdomen Pose** for three minutes on each side.

3. Use one bolster for **Side Lying Stretch**. Focus on taking full breaths in and out. Hold this pose for four minutes per side.

4. Transition to **Child's Pose (Option 2)**. Stay in this pose for ten minutes.

5. Move down to the floor and practice **Cross Bolster Pose** for six minutes.

6. Transition into **Legs on Chair**. Hold for ten minutes.

7. Move into **Savasana** and hold the pose for fifteen minutes. Use the eye pillow, if desired.

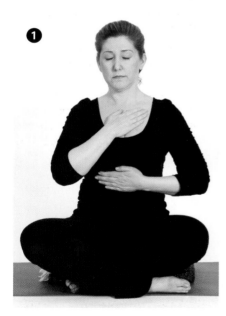

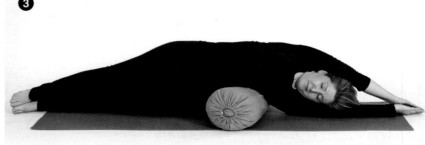

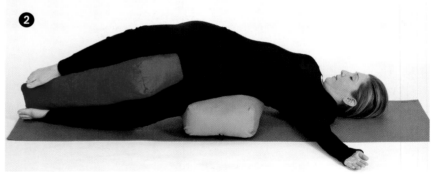

4

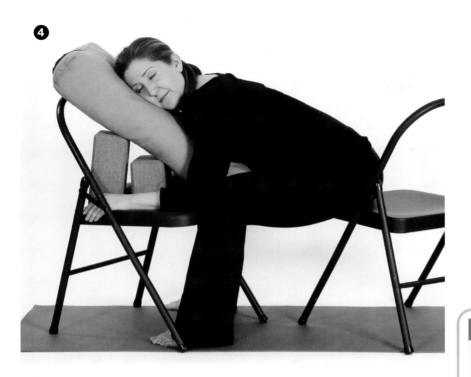

5

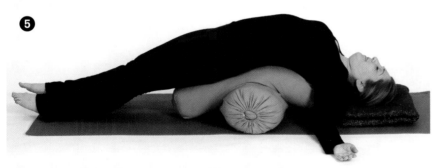

THREADS OF THOUGHT

Ahiṁsā-satya-asteya brahmacarya-aparigrahās yamās

Respect for others (yama) means practicing nonviolence (ahimsa), truthfulness (satya), never stealing (asteya), never comparing yourself to others (aparigraha), and acting from an awareness of higher ideals (brahma-charya).

6

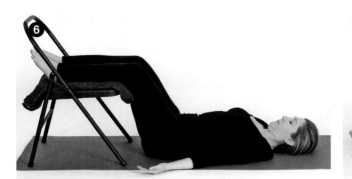

7

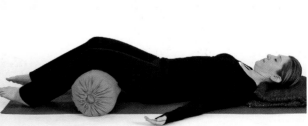

SEQUENCES FOR WOMEN'S ISSUES

Menopause tends to cause discomfort and moodiness, while pregnancy has its own set of discomforts and limitations. Both are good reasons to give restorative yoga a try. Hormonal imbalance is regulated through the practice of restorative yoga in general, and by the sequences in this section in particular. It's a wonderfully calming practice that helps women find ease in their bodies during these challenging times. Practice and enjoy!

MENOPAUSE

TIME: 30 minutes

YOU NEED:
- Mat
- Strap
- 2 blocks
- 1–2 bolsters
- 2 blankets (Rectangle Fold and Square Fold)
- Eye pillow (optional)

Menopause can be a trying time for women. Weight gain, mood swings, forgetfulness, night sweats, hot flashes, and a variety of other symptoms can make women not feel like themselves. Fortunately, restorative yoga can help women cool down: the more relaxed you get, the lower your body temperature drops. It will also calm your nervous system and decrease agitation. Yoga can truly ease the symptoms of menopause, and many women find restorative yoga to be exactly what they need to get through this time.

SHORT SEQUENCE

WHAT TO DO

1. Sit in a comfortable position to practice **Sitali Breath** to cool and center your body for one minute.

2. From here, do three rounds of **Shoulder Stretches** to loosen up the upper body.

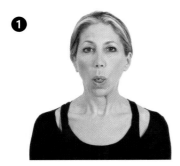

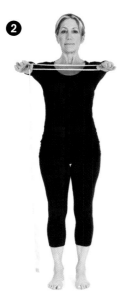

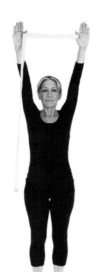

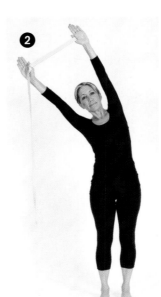

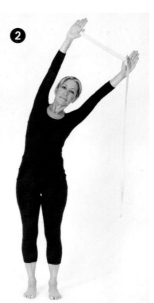

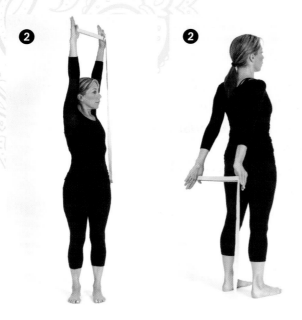

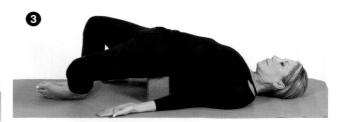

3. Lie back for **Simple Bridge with Block or Bolster under Hips**, using a block for this sequence. Hold the pose for five minutes. Next, bring the soles of your feet together, keeping your knees out to the side. Hold this pose for one minute, then move your legs together, lift your hips, and remove the block. Let your back relax on the floor for three minutes.

4. Set up for **Reclining Hero Pose (Option 2)**. Be sure to use any additional props as needed. Stay here for six minutes.

5. Transition into **Fan Pose** for four minutes.

6. Move into **Savasana** and hold the pose for twelve minutes. Use the eye pillow, if desired.

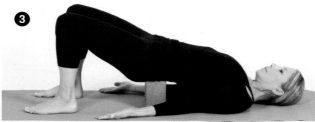

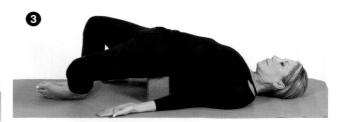

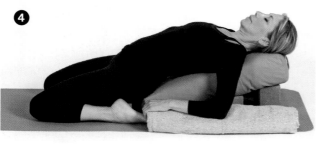

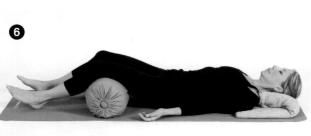

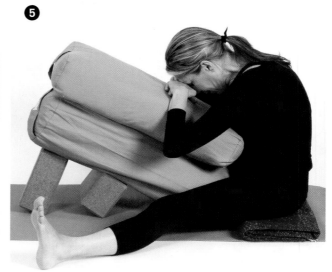

TIME: 1 hour

YOU NEED:
- Mat
- Wall
- Bolster
- 2 blocks
- 2 blankets (Rectangle and Head Rest Fold)
- Eye pillow (optional)

WHAT TO DO

1. Sit in a comfortable position to practice **Sitali Breath** to cool and center yourself for one minute.

2. Move to the wall for **Legs Up the Wall Pose Without Bolster**. Hold the pose for ten minutes.

3. Set up for **Belly Down Twist over Bolster**. Hold the pose for three minutes on each side.

4. Transition into **Supported Bound Angle Pose (Option 5)**. Stay in this pose for twelve minutes.

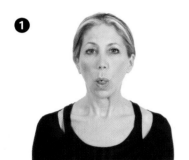

1

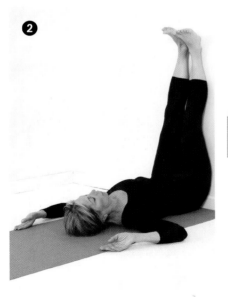

2

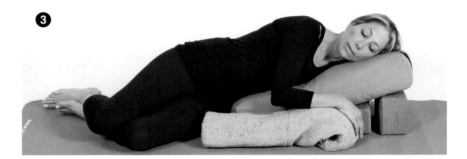

3

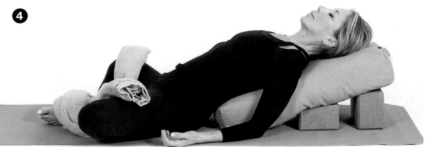

4

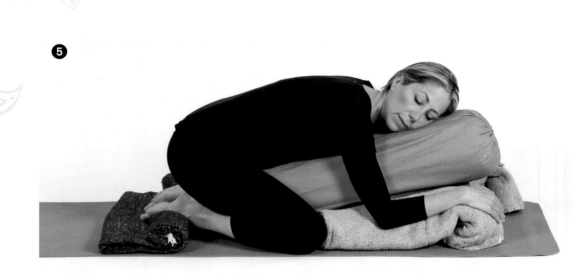

⑤

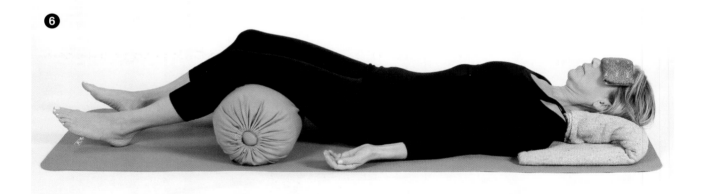

⑥

5. Move into **Child's Pose (Option 1)**. Rest your head to one side for five minutes, then switch to the other side for another five minutes (ten minutes total).

6. Move into **Savasana** and hold the pose for fifteen minutes. Use an eye pillow for relaxation, if desired.

PREGNANCY

Restorative yoga offers a lot to expectant mothers. While women who are pregnant can certainly practice yoga, it becomes more difficult to during the last trimester, when the body becomes challenging to maneuver. Some postures, such as the twists and inversions offered in more active yoga classes, are simply not recommended for women during various stages of pregnancy. Fortunately, because of its gentle nature, restorative yoga is a fantastic practice for pregnant women, and can offer many benefits including reducing discomfort and creating an overall healthy pregnancy experience. It is, by nature, a supportive practice, and pregnant women really benefit from the relaxed feeling that it promotes. The following sequences are designed for women who are in any stage of pregnancy. Make sure to gather extra props before beginning to provide extra support for your belly and back as needed.

TIME: 30 minutes

YOU NEED:
- Mat
- Wall
- Chair
- 2 bolsters
- 2 blocks
- 2 blankets (Square Fold and Rectangle Fold)

SHORT SEQUENCE

WHAT TO DO

1. Move to the wall for **Wall Downward-Facing Dog**. Hold the pose for two minutes.

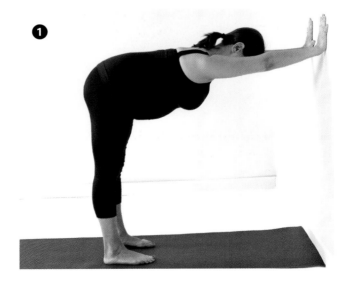

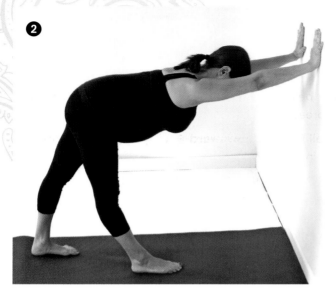

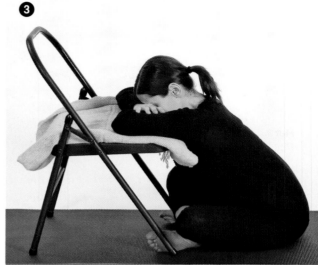

2. Stay at the wall for **Wall Half-Triangle Forward Bend**. Hold for one minute, then switch legs and hold for another minute.

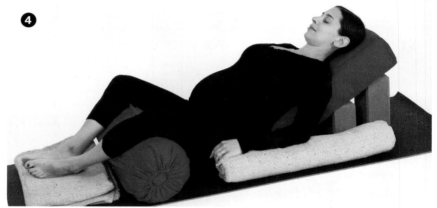

3. Move to a chair for **Chair Forward Bend (Option 1)**. Hold the pose for three minutes, then cross your legs the other way and hold for another three minutes.

4. Move to the floor for **Supported Bound Angle Pose (Option 4)**. Hold the pose for ten minutes.

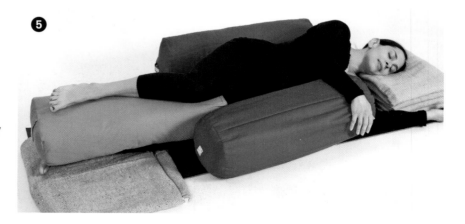

5. Move into **Side Lying Savasana** (on your left side) for ten minutes. Use as many props as necessary to make yourself comfortable.

TIME: 1 hour

YOU NEED:
- Mat
- Wall
- 2 bolsters
- 4 blankets (Square Fold, Head Rest Fold, Small Square Fold)
- 2–4 blocks

WHAT TO DO

1. Center for a few minutes, focusing on your breath with your hands resting on your belly. You can use **Apa Japa Breath** here, or just observe your breathing.

2. Move to the wall for **Wall Downward-Facing Dog**. Stay in this pose for two minutes.

3. Stay at the wall for **Wall Half-Triangle Forward Bend**. Hold for one minute with one foot forward, then switch legs and hold for another minute.

4. Move to the floor for **Belly Down Twist over Bolster**. Hold for three minutes per side.

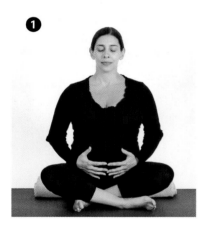

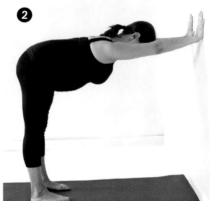

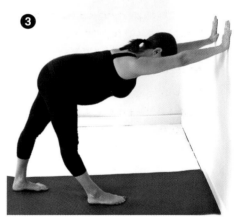

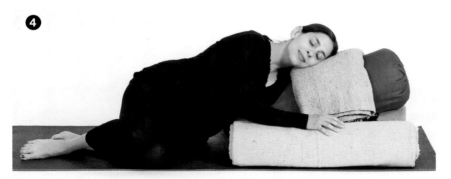

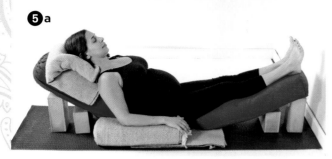

5 a

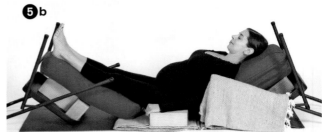

5 b

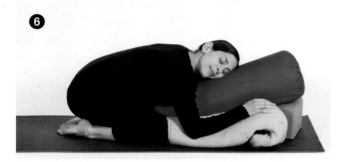

6

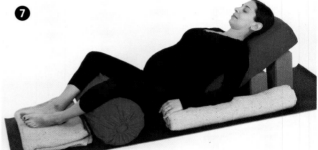

7

5. Set up for **Legs Up the Wall Pose with Bolster** or **Two Chair Boat Pose**. If you decide to do **Legs Up the Wall Pose with Bolster** you will want to be propped up with a bolster on an angle and have your legs propped up on an angled bolster as well. Stay in the pose of your choice for ten minutes.

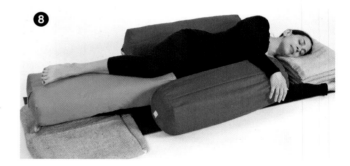

8

6. Move into **Child's Pose (Option 1)** and rest in the pose for ten minutes.

7. Relax in **Supported Bound Angle Pose (Option 4)** for ten minutes.

8. Finish up with **Side Lying Savasana** (on your left side) for ten minutes. Use as many props as necessary to make yourself comfortable.

•

YOGIC WISDOM

The following are not recommended for pregnant women practicing yoga:

• *Do not lie on right side or on your belly after first trimester.*

• *Do not lie flat on your back after first trimester.*

• *Avoid overstretching.*

• *Do not hold your breath in any breathing practices.*

SEQUENCES FOR OTHER HEALTH ISSUES

Dis-ease is created when there is a lack of harmony in the body. Whether you're suffering from insomnia or cancer, if you do not feel at ease in your body, certain conditions can arise. The restorative yoga sequences in this section are not only helpful in treating these and other common health problems, but also helpful in preventing them.

INSOMNIA

Do you often have trouble falling or staying asleep? Insomnia is caused by a variety of health issues, including chronic pain, menopause, depression, anxiety, heartburn, and others. But even though a variety of issues can cause insomnia, the root cause of this issue is overstimulation of the nervous system, caused by stress. Restorative yoga is the perfect antidote: It helps ground you, which relaxes the nervous system and helps promote a restful body. The following sequences are designed to ground you in your body through your breath first, and then through the weight of sandbags as you lie fully relaxed on the floor. If any pose stimulates you too much, feel free to remove it from the sequence.

TIME: 30 minutes

YOU NEED:
- Mat
- Bolster
- Sandbag
- Blanket (Rectangle Fold) (optional)
- Eye pillow (optional)

SHORT SEQUENCE

WHAT TO DO

1. Begin with **Ujjaii Breath (Option 1)** to begin to slow down the brain. Remember this is a "loud" breath, so you should be able to hear it as you constrict your throat. Practice this breathing for two minutes.

2. Next, place a bolster on the floor for **Down Dog with Head on Block or Bolster**, using a bolster for this particular sequence. Hold for two minutes.

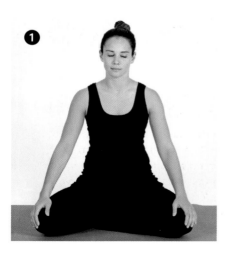

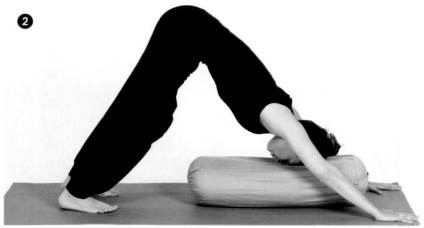

3. Move into **Side Lying Stretch**. Hold the pose for three minutes on each side. Let your body relax fully over the bolster, using your bottom arm as a pillow for your head.

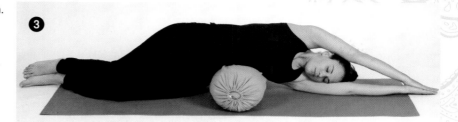

4. Now transition to your belly for **Belly Down with Bolster at Hip**. Let your belly fully relax over the bolster. Hold the pose for three minutes.

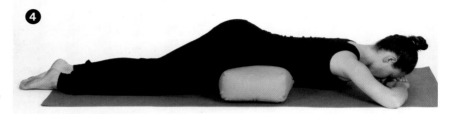

5. Press back into **Child's Pose (Option 1)**. For this sequence, place a sandbag on your back. Relax in this pose for seven minutes as you feel the pressure of the sandbag on your back.

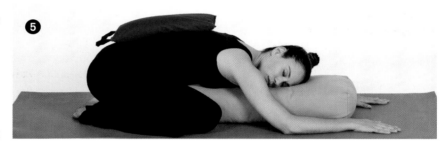

6. Finally, move into **Savasana**. For this sequence, place a sandbag on your chest, and let the weight of the sandbag dissolve any remaining tension. Hold the pose for ten minutes. Add an eye pillow and/or blanket to help you relax even further, if you like.

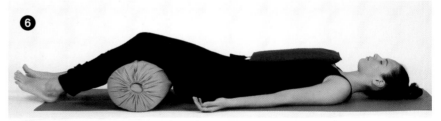

YOGIC WISDOM

In Ayurveda, the day can be divided into a "body clock" organized by the doshas. According to the doshic energy that is dominant at that time of day, some times are best for eating, some for thinking, some for exercising, and some for resting. According to Ayurvedic wisdom, the best times to sleep are 10:00 P.M. to 2:00 A.M., when Pitta helps you "digest" your thoughts and food from the day, and from 2:00 A.M. to 6:00 A.M., when Vata moves and helps you eliminate the byproducts of digestion. Sleeping during these times will help you maintain your body's internal clock.

TIME: 1 hour

YOU NEED:

- Mat
- Chair
- Bolster
- 2 blocks (optional)
- Wall
- Sandbag
- Blanket (Head Rest Fold or Rectangle Fold) (optional)
- Eye pillow (optional)

WHAT TO DO

1. Attune to your breath for a few minutes using **Ujjaii Breath (Option 2)**, which increases the length of your exhalation.

2. Transition to **Down Dog with Head on Block or Bolster**, using a bolster for this particular sequence. Hold the pose for two minutes.

3. Lower to your knees and come into **Child's Pose (Option 1)**. Hold the pose for eight minutes.

4. Rise to move into **Chair Forward Bend (Option 1)**. Make sure to use any props necessary to support your seat or your legs to avoid any discomfort in your hips or knees. Hold the pose for four minutes, then switch your legs and hold for another four minutes.

5. Lie on a bolster for **Supported Bound Angle Pose (Option 1)**. If needed, use a Head Rest Fold blanket on top of the bolster to support your head, and blocks to support your thighs. Hold for twelve minutes.

6. Move to a wall for **Legs Up the Wall Without Bolster**. Place a sandbag across the soles of your feet. Hold the pose for ten minutes.

7. Move into **Side Lying Savasana**. Use as many props as you need to make yourself comfortable. Hold the pose for fifteen minutes.

❶

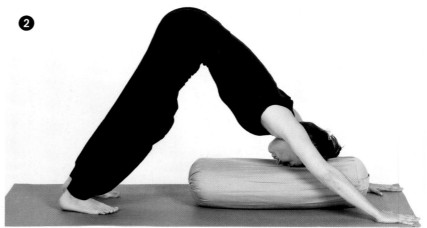

❷

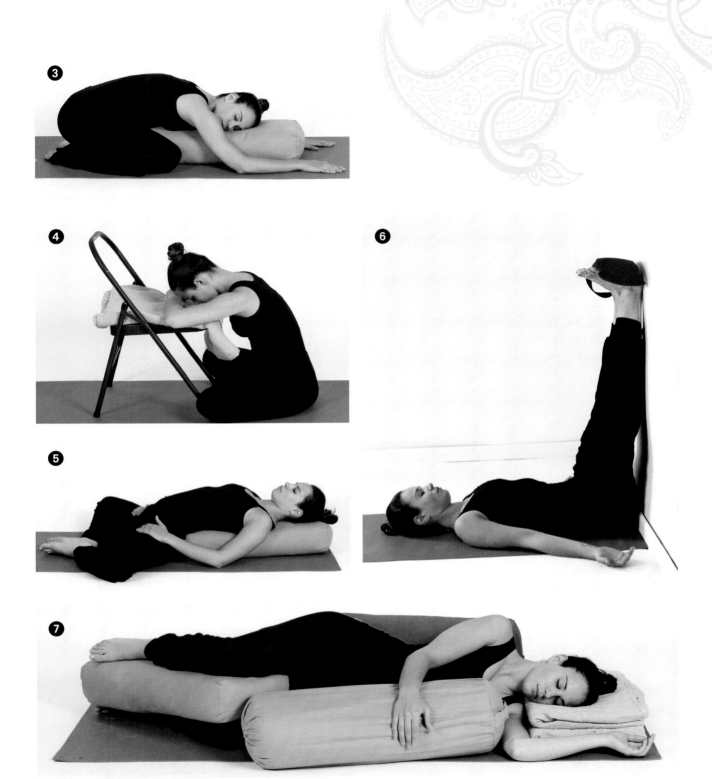

HEADACHES

Headaches can be caused by tension in the muscles of the head and neck, from allergic reactions, from sinus pressure, colds, flu—the list is long. One of the major sources of headaches is stress, which is where restorative yoga can really help. Think of your neck muscles like a vise. If the vise grips, blood cannot flow well to the brain. If you relax your neck and its supporting muscles you release that grip. The following sequences include postures and breathing exercises that will help you bring awareness to your body to release tension and ease your headache pain.

TIME: 30 minutes

YOU NEED:
- Mat
- Strap
- Bolster
- 2 blocks
- 2 blankets (Long Roll Fold)
- Headwrap

SHORT SEQUENCE

WHAT TO DO

1. Begin this sequence with **Neck Stretches**. Make sure you hold the stretch on each side for at least a couple of breaths, and lengthen the stretch if you can by stretching your arms out to the floor—you want to really feel a full release in your neck area.

2. Next, practice **Shoulder Stretches** for a few minutes.

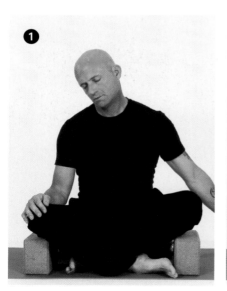

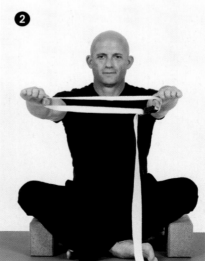

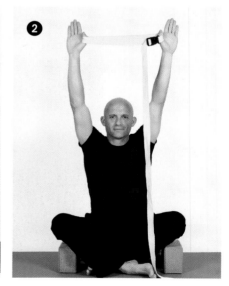

3. Move to the floor for **Fish Pose with Blocks or Bolster**. For this version, use both the blocks and bolster to support you. Wrap your head with a headwrap and hold the pose for ten minutes.

4. Transition to **Supported Bound Angle Pose (Option 1)**. If you feel too much of a stretch, make sure you feel supported under your legs by adding blocks or blankets. Hold for four minutes.

5. Set up for Savasana, using a bolster under your knees. While in this pose, practice the **Cloud** visualization for ten minutes. You will notice fewer thoughts as time goes by.

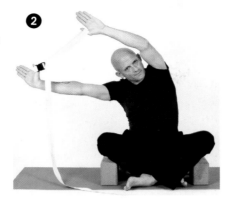

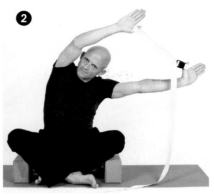

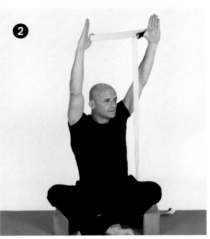

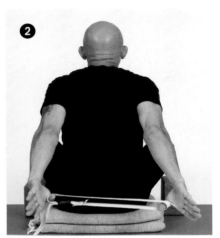

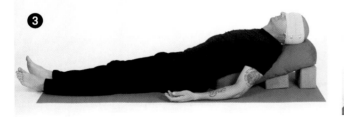

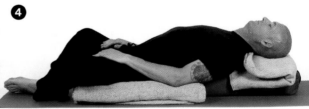

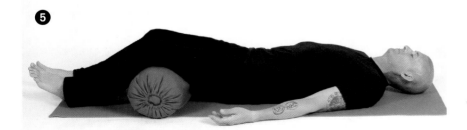

TIME: 1 hour

YOU NEED:
- Mat
- Strap
- Wall
- Chair
- 2 bolsters
- 1–2 blankets (Square Fold and Rectangle Fold)
- Block
- Eye pillow (optional)
- Sandbag

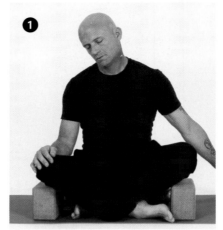

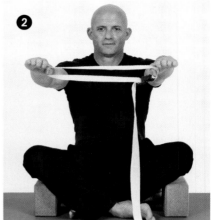

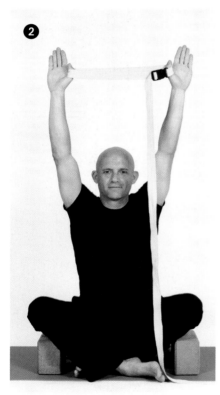

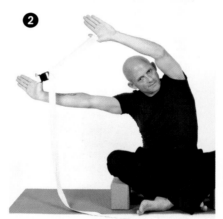

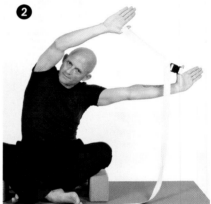

WHAT TO DO

1. Begin this sequence with **Neck Stretches**. Make sure you hold the stretch on each side for at least a couple breaths, and lengthen it if you can by stretching your arms out to the floor—you want to really feel a full release in your neck area.

2. Next, practice **Shoulder Stretches** for a few minutes.

3. Move to a comfortable seated position on the floor and practice **Breath with Pause**. Focus on your breath, pausing briefly after exhaling. Do this for about three minutes.

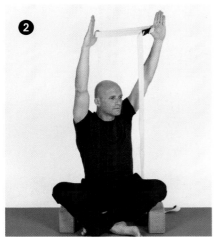

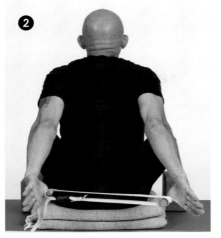

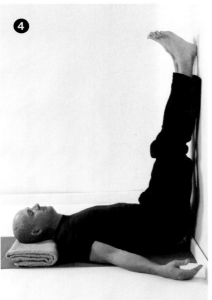

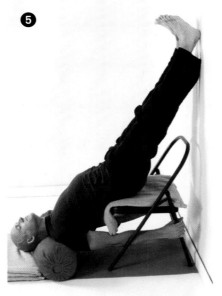

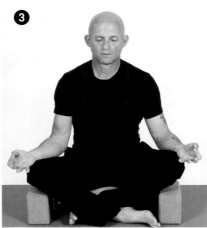

4. Come to the wall for **Legs Up the Wall Pose Without Bolster**. Hold for approximately ten minutes.

5. Roll to your side and take a moment to adjust before moving into **Chair Shoulder Stand**. Settle into this pose and hold for about six minutes, then lower yourself down so that your lower back rests on the bolster and your legs rest on the chair. Hold this pose for one minute before you move on.

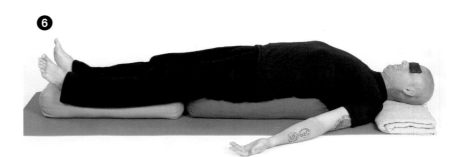

6. Set up for **Reclining Bridge Pose (Option 1)** with your bolsters and any blankets you might need. Use an eye pillow for relaxation, if desired. Hold for eight minutes.

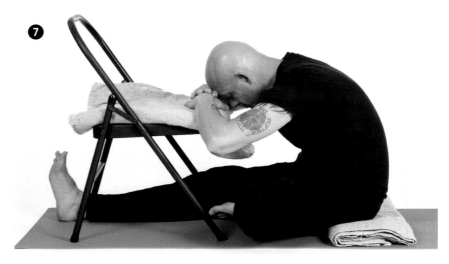

7. Come to your chair for **Chair Forward Bend (Option 2)**. Hold for three minutes on each leg. Remember to prop up your leg with a blanket or block if you have any discomfort in your hip or knee.

8. Move into **Belly Down Twist over Bolster** and hold for three minutes on each side. It's okay to turn your head toward or away from your knees for a deeper twist, but be mindful not to force it. Remain comfortable.

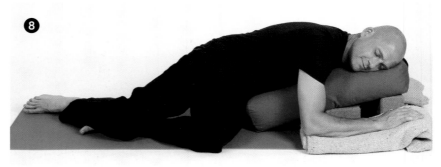

9. Finally, move to **Savasana**. For this sequence, place a sandbag on your forehead. Prop up the sandbag so that it rests partially on your forehead and partially on a block above your head. Hold the pose for fifteen minutes. Be mindful when you remove the sandbag to avoid any strain.

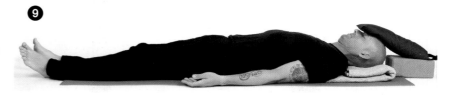

CANCER

With medications, surgeries, and the stress of prognoses, it is easy for cancer sufferers to feel overwhelmed in both mind and body. Perhaps one of the most beneficial effects of restorative yoga is that it helps these people deepen the awareness of their bodies and become aware of their different bodily functions. Developing this mind/body connection can actually be an astonishingly beneficial tool in helping cancer sufferers regain a sense of control over their health. Specifically, restorative yoga's effect on the lymphatic system can be especially helpful in stimulating the body's healing processes when dealing with cancer. The following sequences can help aid your body in fighting the disease, as well as aid you in recovery.

TIME: 30 minutes

YOU NEED:
- Mat
- Strap
- 2 blankets (Long Roll Fold, Square Fold, Rectangle Fold, Open Fold)
- Chair
- Wall
- Bolster
- Eye pillow (optional)

SHORT SEQUENCE

WHAT TO DO

1. Practice **Apa Japa Breath** for about two minutes to center yourself.

2. Then practice **Shoulder Stretches** for about four minutes. Be mindful not to overstretch.

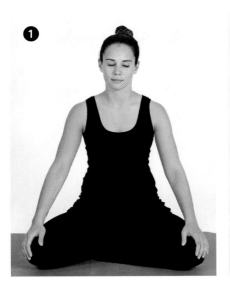
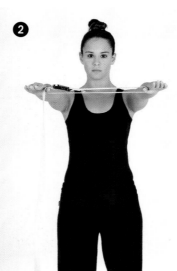
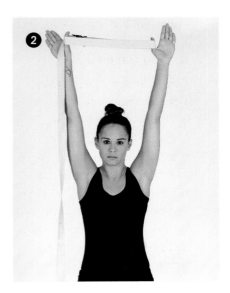

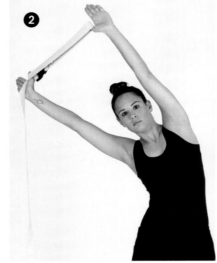

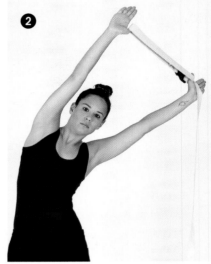

3. Then take two minutes in each position in **Blanket Roll in 3 Positions**, for a total of six minutes.

4. Set up your chair for **Chair Forward Bend (Option 1)**. Hold the position for three minutes, then switch your legs and hold for another three minutes.

5. Move to the wall for **Legs Up the Wall Pose with Bolster**. Place the bolster under your hips and a Rectangle Fold blanket under your back. Hold for five minutes.

6. Move into **Savasana** and hold the pose for about ten minutes. An extra blanket in an Open Fold and an eye pillow are good here.

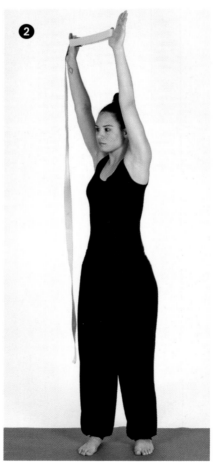

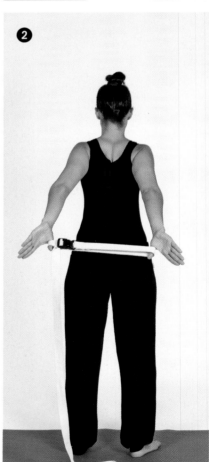

3

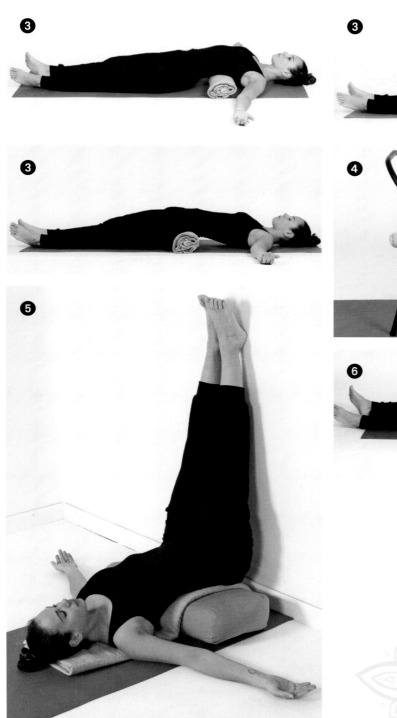

3

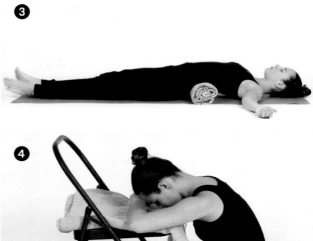

3

4

5

6

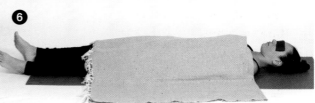

YOU NEED:

- Mat
- Wall
- 2 bolsters
- 2 chairs
- 2–4 blankets (Half Fold, Head Rest Fold, Square Fold, Rectangle Fold)
- 4 blocks
- Eye pillow (optional)

LONG SEQUENCE

WHAT TO DO

1. Begin by practicing **Apa Japa Breath**. As you breathe, practice the **White Light** visualization from Chapter 4 for about five minutes.

2. Next practice **Wall Half-Triangle Forward Bend**. Hold the pose for four minutes.

3. Come down to set up for **Supported Bound Angle Pose (Option 4)**. Use one bolster angled over two blocks under your back, and one bolster under your knees. Wrap a blanket around you so you are swaddled. Stay in this pose for ten minutes or more.

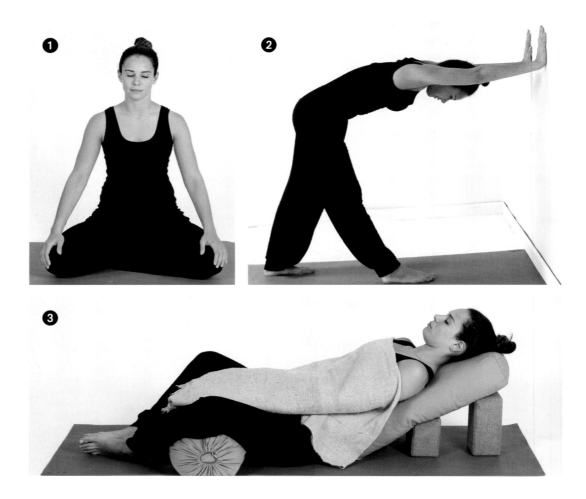

4. Move on to **Heart Opening Pose**. Be sure to prop your neck if you need the support. Hold this pose for ten minutes.

5. Come into **Chair Forward Bend (Option 1)**. Sit cross-legged for three minutes on each side.

6. With the second chair, set up for **Two Chair Boat Pose**. Stay in this pose for ten minutes.

7. Move into **Savasana**. While in this pose, focus on relaxing each part of your body methodically with the **Yoga Nidra** visualization in Chapter 4. Stay in this pose for fifteen minutes or more. If desired, cover yourself with a blanket and use an eye pillow for added relaxation.

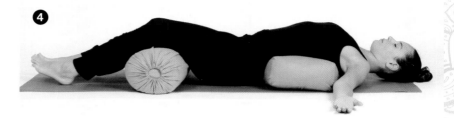

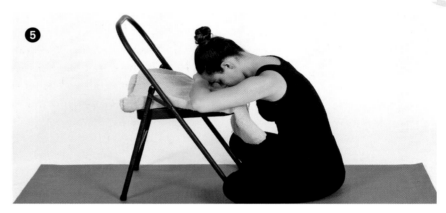

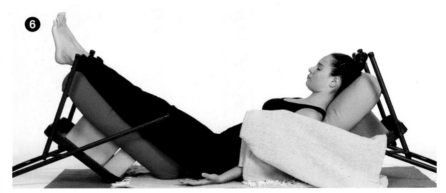

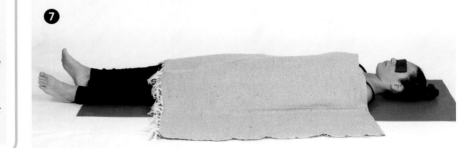

YOGIC WISDOM

Do not overdo it. If you are tired, listen to your body and do fewer poses, held for less time. The idea is to maintain mindfulness about not pushing yourself, and easing back into your body's movements. Also, do not practice any yoga for at least two weeks after surgery.

OSTEOPOROSIS AND OSTEOPENIA

TIME: 30 minutes

YOU NEED:
- Mat
- 2 bolsters
- Sandbag
- Blanket (Head Rest Fold)
- Eye pillow (optional)

One of the best ways restorative yoga helps those with osteoporosis and osteopenia is by reducing tension in the body. While it is well known that weight-bearing exercises help build bone density and slow the progression of the disease, we are also beginning to understand that reducing cortisol levels in the body is also helpful in slowing the process of osteoporosis, as high cortisol levels can exacerbate bone density loss. The following sequences will help you to reduce tension in the body, thereby reducing cortisol production. Restorative yoga can also help those with osteoporosis by creating mindfulness, which can be an important factor in those suffering from the disease. When you are more mindful in general, you become more mindful of your body and your surroundings, which can reduce your chances of falling and injury. And, of course, restorative yoga offers an option to those who cannot practice a more vigorous style of yoga. The poses here are very gentle on the body, but, as always, do not push yourself. The point is to stay relaxed and to reduce tension in the body.

SHORT SEQUENCE

WHAT TO DO

1. Begin in **Reclining Bridge Pose (Option 1)**. Hold the pose for ten minutes.

2. Come into **Child's Pose (Option 1)**. For this sequence, place a sandbag on your back. Sometimes it's difficult to get it on just right; if you have a friend to help you, that is great. Stay in this pose for ten minutes.

3. Move to the floor for **Savasana**. For this specific sequence, place a sandbag on your abdomen. Stay in this pose for ten minutes. Use a blanket and an eye pillow for extra relaxation, if you like.

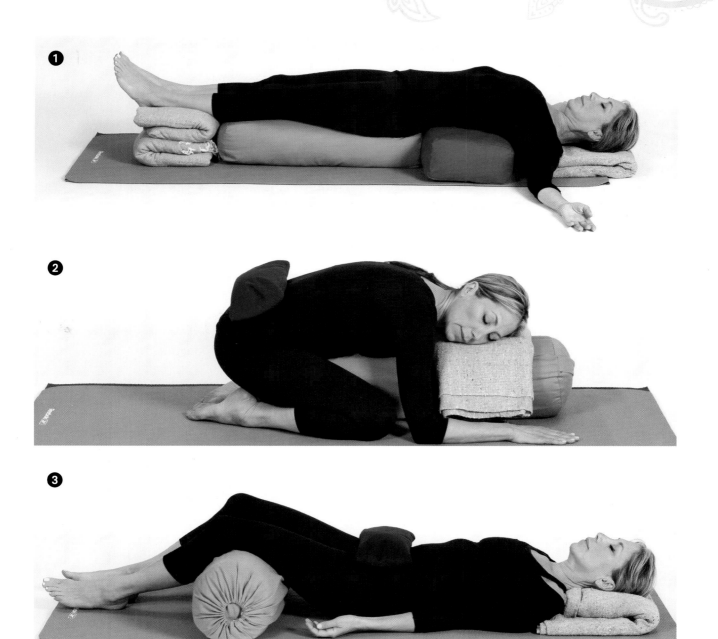

TIME: 1 hour

YOU NEED:
- Mat
- Wall
- 2 bolsters
- 2 blocks
- Sandbag
- 2 blankets (Head Rest Fold and Rectangle Fold)
- Eye pillow (optional)

WHAT TO DO

1. Begin with **Wall Downward-Facing Dog**. Hold this pose for four minutes.

2. Stay at the wall for **Wall Half-Triangle Forward Bend**. Spend two minutes on each side.

3. Move to the floor for **Legs Up the Wall Pose Without Bolster**. Place a sandbag across the soles of your feet, and hold this pose for ten minutes. When you come out of the pose, be mindful when taking the sandbag off, to avoid causing any strain.

4. Move into **Child's Pose (Option 1)**. For this sequence, place a sandbag on your back. Stay in this pose for ten minutes.

5. Transition to **Side Lying Stretch**. Use one bolster. Hold the pose on your right side for four minutes, and then move to your left side and hold for four minutes more.

6. Roll onto your belly for **Belly Down with Bolster at Hip**. Stay in this pose for eight minutes.

7. Finally, rest in **Savasana**. For this particular sequence, place a sandbag on your abdomen. Hold for at least fifteen minutes for deep relaxation. Use an eye pillow, if you like.

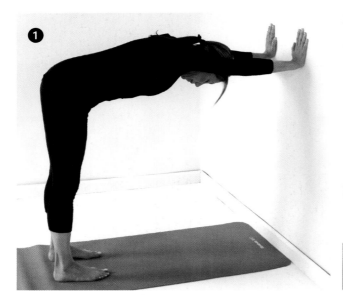

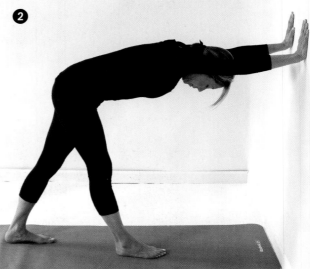

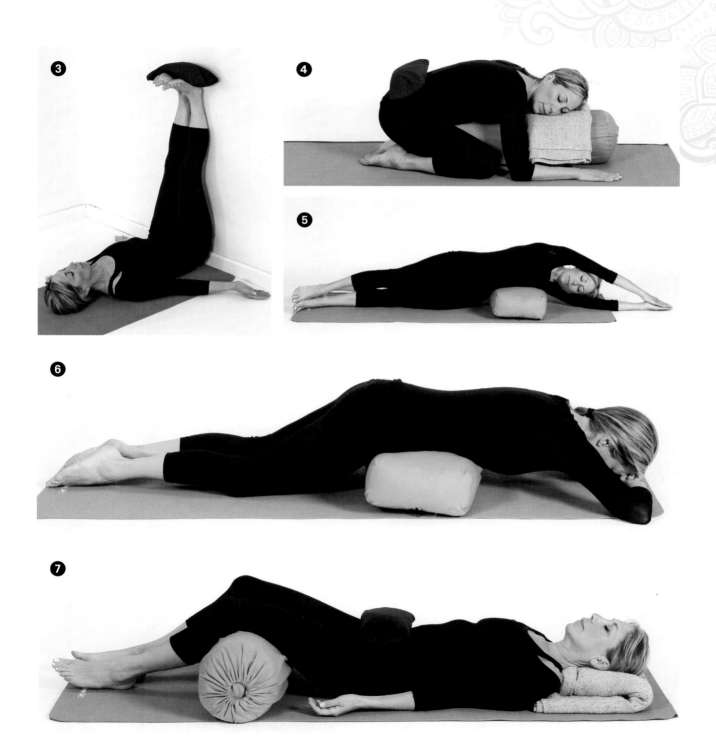

JET LAG

TIME: 40 minutes

YOU NEED:
- Mat
- Strap
- Chair
- 2 bolsters
- 2 blankets (Square Fold and Rectangle Fold)
- Eye pillow (optional)

If you travel often by plane, you know the troubles that can come with air travel. Your body becomes compressed by sitting in cramped seats for long periods of time, and you come off the plane with aches, pains, and even digestive upset. Additionally, travel across time zones can interfere with your internal body clock and wreak havoc on your sleep. Thankfully, restorative yoga can help you get your sleep rhythms back in place, release and open up tension in the body, and get back to business. The following sequences focus on stretching and opening those areas of the body that become crunched and collapsed during travel, and focus on making you feel grounded.
You can find any of the props you need for the following poses in any standard hotel room (improvise if necessary!).

SHORT SEQUENCE

WHAT TO DO

1. Begin with **Shoulder Stretches** for a few minutes. (It's always helpful to stretch your shoulders right away after travel.)

2. Move to a chair for **Chair Forward Bend (Option 2)**. Sit for six minutes before switching legs, then sit for another six minutes.

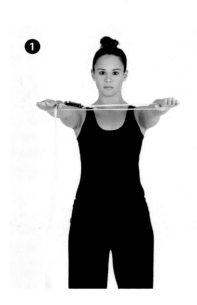

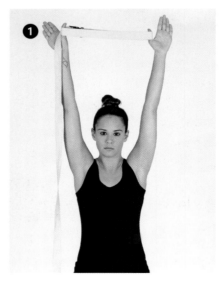

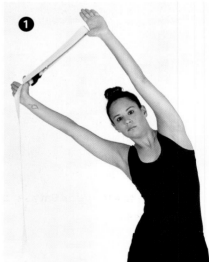

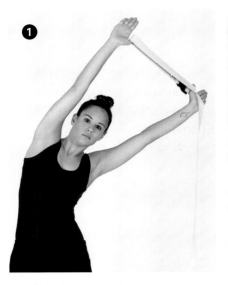
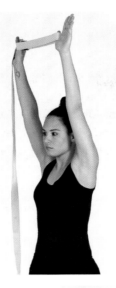
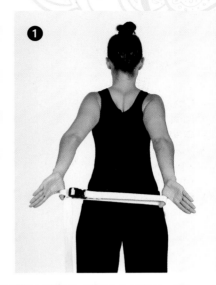

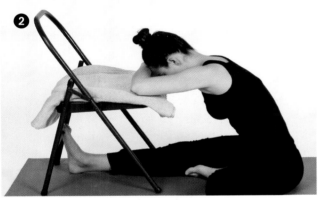

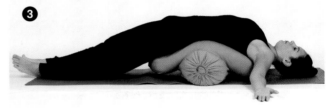

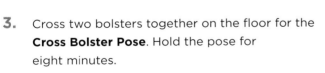

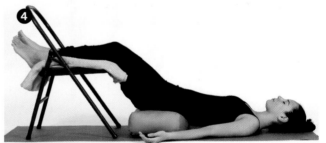

3. Cross two bolsters together on the floor for the **Cross Bolster Pose**. Hold the pose for eight minutes.

4. Set up for **Legs on Chair**. Be sure to place a bolster under your hips. Hold the pose for ten minutes to release any lingering tension in your hips and pelvis.

5. Lie on the floor for **Savasana**. Stay for ten minutes.

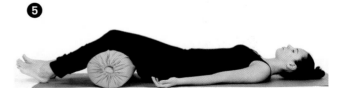

TIME: 1 hour

YOU NEED:
- Mat
- Wall
- Bolster
- 2 blankets (Accordion Fold)
- Strap
- 2 blocks
- Sandbag (optional)
- Eye pillow (optional)

WHAT TO DO

1. Move to a wall for **Legs Up the Wall Pose Without Bolster**. Hold the pose for twelve minutes.

2. Move into **Supported Bound Angle Pose (Option 3)**. Hold for ten minutes.

3. Move into **Scissored Legs Belly Down Twist**. Hold for three minutes on each side.

4. Transition into **Pigeon Pose with Bolster**. Hold the pose for six minutes, then shift legs and hold for another six minutes.

5. Come to **Seated Twist (Option 1)**. Try to focus on taking full breaths in, and fully exhaling as you come into the twist. When you are in the twist, take at least three breaths in and out on each side.

6. Move into **Savasana**. Hold the pose for fifteen minutes. Add a sandbag to your belly for a greater sense of grounding. Use an eye pillow, if desired.

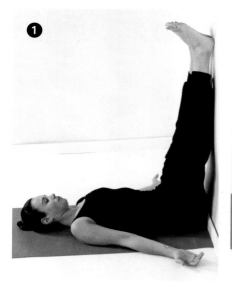

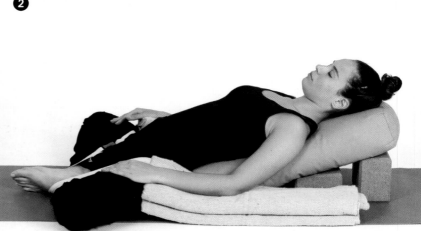

③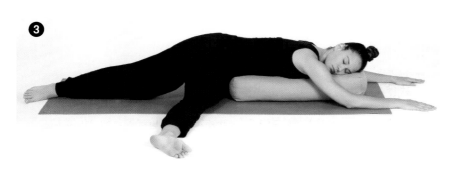

④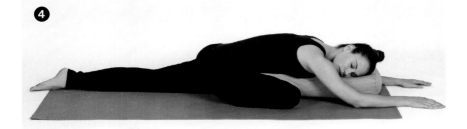

⑤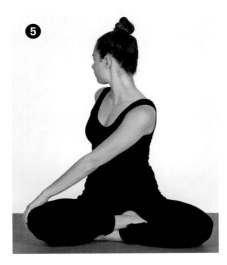

⑥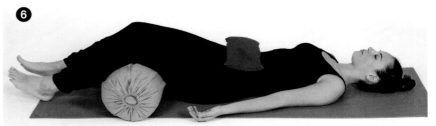

SORE MUSCLES

Weekend warriors—you know who you are. On the weekends, you're the one going for a 7:00 A.M. run or spin class, followed by an afternoon basketball game, maybe a round of golf with friends squeezed in, and any number of other activities. Sure, your body is happy with the exercise, but it has a way of rebelling if you overdo it. As we get older, recovery from these activities gets more difficult, and can last all the way into midweek. Fortunately, restorative yoga will bring your tired, sore muscles back to life and help you stay a warrior. This following short restorative yoga sequence can be done on weekdays, and the longer session saved for the weekend.

TIME: 40 minutes

YOU NEED:

- Mat
- Bolster
- 2 blankets (Oblong Fold, Head Rest Fold, Rectangle Fold)
- Wall
- 2 blocks
- Eye pillow (optional)

SHORT SEQUENCE

WHAT TO DO

1. Begin with **Supported Bound Angle Pose (Option 5)**. Hold the pose for ten minutes.

2. Come to the wall for **Legs Up the Wall Pose with Bolster**. Stay in the pose for ten minutes. Feel the blood flow back down your legs.

3. Rest in **Child's Pose (Option 1)** for six minutes.

4. Next move into **Belly Down Twist over Bolster**. Hold for three minutes on each side.

5. Finally, come to **Savasana**, placing a bolster under your knees. Stay in the pose for ten minutes. Use an eye pillow, if desired.

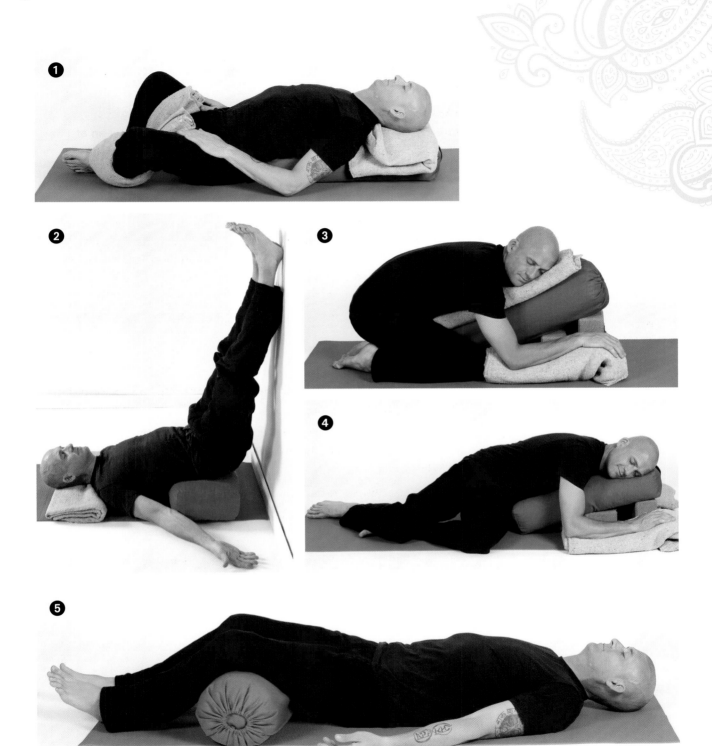

TIME: 1 hour

YOU NEED:
- Mat
- Wall
- Strap
- 3 blankets (Rectangle Fold, Long Roll Fold, Small Square Fold)
- 2 bolsters
- 2 blocks
- Eye pillow (optional)

WHAT TO DO

1. Begin with **Cat/Cow Tilts with Feet on Wall** focusing on inhaling when you are in Cow, and exhaling when you shift to Cat. Do this for about two minutes.

2. Take your strap and move to **Extended Hand to Foot Pose, Supine**. While lying on your back, hold each leg up, out to the side, and across your body for one minute each before switching legs.

3. Sit for **Shoulder Stretches**, doing one round of each of the stretches in the series.

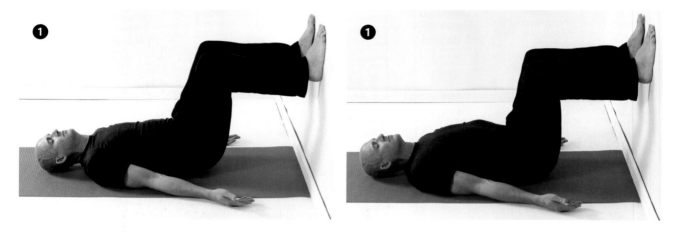

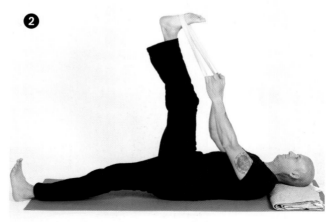

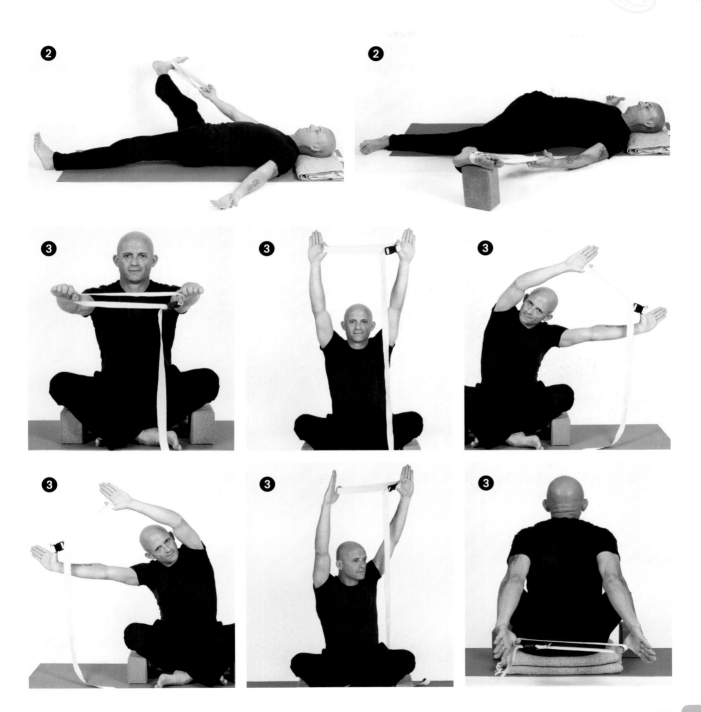

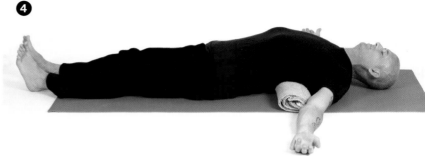

4. Lie down for **Blanket Roll in 3 Positions**. Stay in each position for two minutes.

5. Move into **Supported Bound Angle Pose (Option 1)** with a blanket rolled under each leg. You may find you need a blanket under your head as well. Stay in this pose for ten minutes.

6. Move into **Revolved Abdomen Pose**. Hold for three minutes on each side.

7. Shift to **Fan Pose** and hold it for six minutes. Feel free to use as many props as needed for comfort.

8. Transition to **Legs Up the Wall Pose with Bolster**. Hold the pose for ten minutes.

9. Lie down on the floor for **Savasana**. You may want to support your legs with a bolster and a strap around your legs if you overdid it this weekend! Use an eye pillow for relaxation, if desired. Stay in the pose for ten minutes.

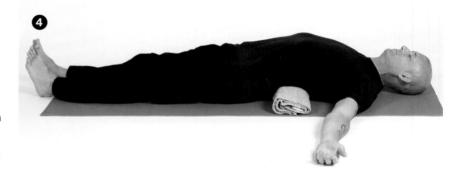

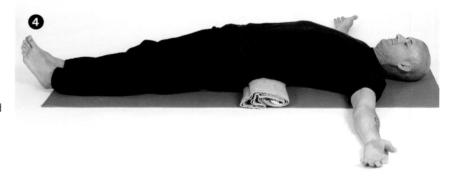

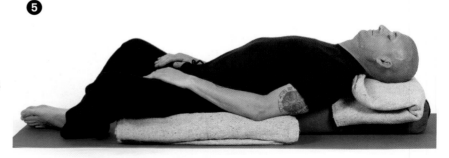

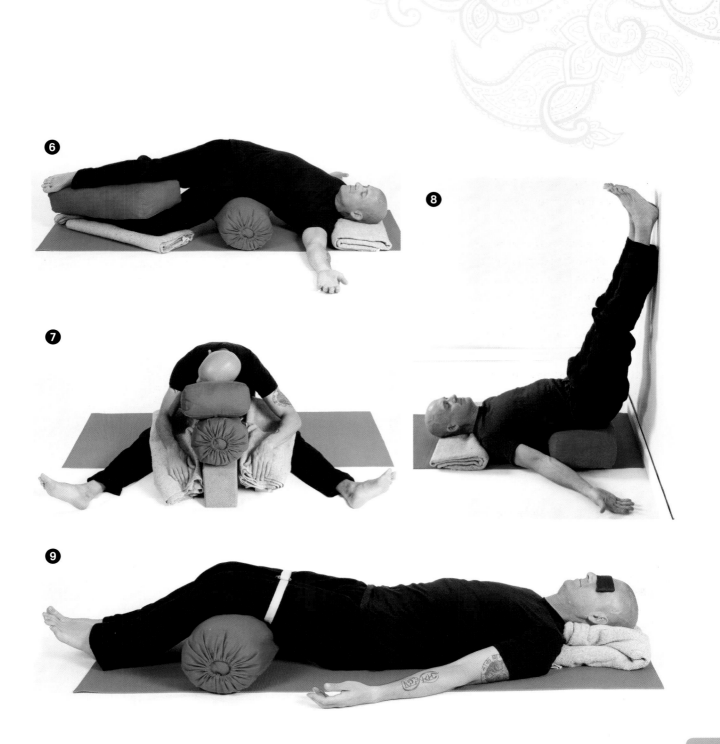

WEIGHT LOSS

More and more people are falling prey to stress in our fast-paced society, and gaining weight as a result. When we become stressed, the fight-or-flight syndrome triggers a complex shift in hormones designed to draw on energy sources quickly in response, which can cause your appetite to increase in order to replenish that energy. You begin to eat when you aren't really hungry or in need of food. Fortunately, restorative yoga can help you lose weight, as it helps reduce stress and rebalance your body's hormonal system. Restorative yoga also creates mindfulness, which will help you curb your appetite and take control of your choices in general. The following sequences are designed to reduce stress and stimulate the digestive system. Best of all, they are available to everyone, regardless of body type.

TIME: 30 minutes

YOU NEED:
- Mat
- 2 blankets (Small Square Fold, Long Roll Fold, Square Fold, Head Rest Fold)
- Chair
- Eye pillow (optional)

SHORT SEQUENCE

WHAT TO DO

1. Begin with **Breath with Pause**. Practice this for about five minutes.

2. Move into **Blanket Roll in 3 Positions**. Stay in each position for two minutes.

3. Come to a chair for **Chair Forward Bend (Option 1)**. Hold for six minutes on each side.

4. Shift into **Legs on Chair**. Relax in this pose for about twelve minutes.

5. Lie down on the floor for **Savasana**. You can place an eye pillow on your eyes for a deeper sense of relaxation, if desired.

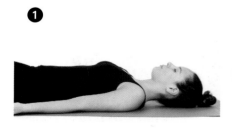

❶

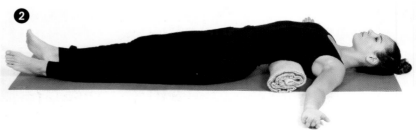

❷

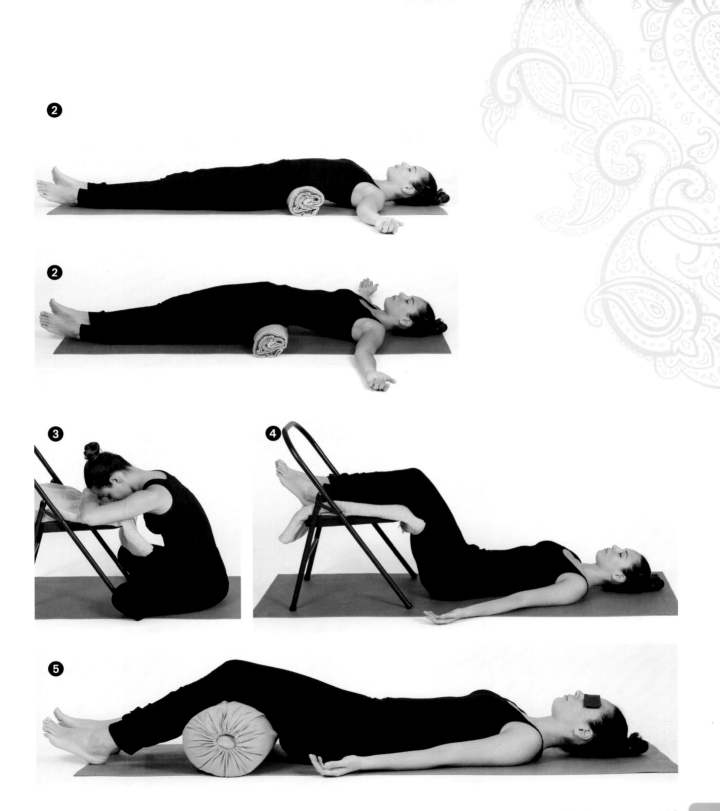

TIME: 1 hour

YOU NEED:

- Mat
- Wall
- 2 blankets (Small Square Fold)
- 2 bolsters
- 2 blocks (optional)
- Eye pillow (optional)

WHAT TO DO

1. Begin with **Breath with Pause**. Practice this for about five minutes.

2. Transition to **Wall Half-Triangle Forward Bend**. Hold for two minutes on each side.

3. Shift into **Fish Pose with Blocks or Bolster**. Hold for eight minutes.

4. Move into **Belly Down Twist over Bolster**. Spend three minutes on each side.

5. Move to **Legs Up the Wall Pose with Bolster**. Stay in the pose for ten minutes.

6. Move into **Side Lying Savasana**. Stay in the posture for about fifteen minutes. Use an eye pillow for deeper relaxation, if desired.

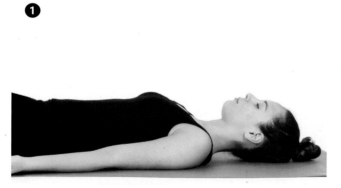

❶

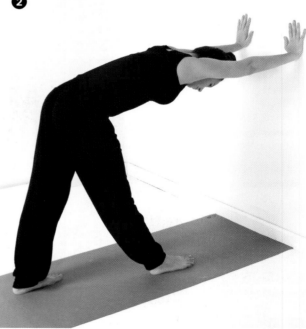

❷

❸

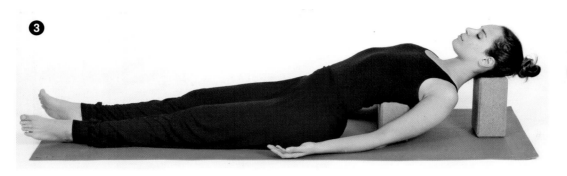

❹

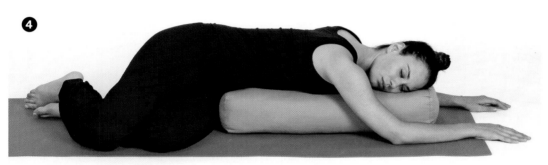

❺

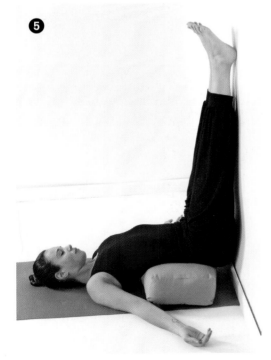

❻

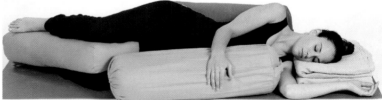

WHERE TO GO FROM HERE

*"There is more wisdom in your body
than in your deepest philosophy."*

—Nietzsche, German philosopher

You've seen the poses, you've seen the sequences. You hopefully have worked with them a bit, and had a chance to understand what restorative yoga is all about. Now what?

If you want to incorporate restorative yoga into your life, the concept of how to sequence a session may be daunting, but it is something that you can do at home. It is my hope that after you have had a chance to work with the poses and sequences, you will have discovered that certain poses really resonate with your body and mind. Combine these poses to form sequences that further resonate with you.

Here are a few pointers that will help you to explore on your own:

- Begin where you are comfortable.

- Practice what feels good for your body, not only while you are in it, but also afterwards, as there is a resonance left from practicing the postures.

- For a practice that has no particular focus, but will leave you feeling great, include:

  - One back bend
  - One twist
  - One forward bend
  - One inversion
  - Savasana

You can't go wrong choosing one from each category.

- Prop yourself up! Use as many props as you need so the pose works for you. Start with the basics and go from there.

- Never stay in a pose if it is uncomfortable; adjust yourself accordingly. If there is discomfort, you won't be able to relax. There is a pose or a variation for everyone; sometimes it means using fewer props, sometimes it means using more. Sometimes it means you cannot be in a certain posture because of an issue you are dealing with. In this case, choose a pose that is from the same category, but may feel more comfortable to maintain if necessary. Know that comfort in restorative yoga is of utmost importance.

- Stay in the pose long enough so that relaxation can set in.

So that's it, in a nutshell. Experiment with the sequences, adjust and swap out poses from the book that you like. Most importantly, show up at your mat as much as you can!

THREADS OF THOUGHT

Abhyasa vairagya abhyam tan nirodhah

The state of yoga is attained through a balance of persistent practice (abhyasa) and nonattachment (vairagya).

RECOMMENDED READING

Following is a list of recommended books for further reading on the topics covered in this book. Included are books on general yoga, books on the philosophies behind yoga, and books that delve more deeply into the restorative yoga practice.

Relax and Renew by Judith Hanson Lasater

The Relaxation Response by Dr. Herbert Benson

American Veda: From Emerson and the Beatles to Yoga and Meditation: How Indian Spirituality Changed the West by Philip Goldberg

Yoga for Emotional Balance: Simple Practices to Help Relieve Anxiety and Depression by Bo Forbes

Yoga for Pain Relief by Kelly McGonigal

Yoga As Medicine by Timothy McCall

Health Through Yoga: Simple Practice Routines and a Guide to the Ancient Teachings by Mira Mehta

The Breathing Book: Good Health and Vitality Through Essential Breath Work by Donna Farhi

The Yoga Sutras of Patanjali by Sri Swami Satchidananda

Tantra Illuminated: The Philosophy, History, and Practice of a Timeless Tradition by Christopher Wallis

The Tree of Yoga by B.K.S. Iyengar

Tantra: The Path of Ecstasy by Georg Feuerstein

Tantra: Cult of the Feminine by Andre van Lysebeth

ACKNOWLEDGMENTS

It's hard to remember a time in my life when I did not feel supported to follow the path my life has taken me on.

I am so grateful to my father, by whom I have been guided my entire life to do what I love. He has been a guide, a mentor, and a wonderful parent. Words could never express how much I love and value you.

To my husband Steven, who is my rock, my cheerleader, my confidant, and best friend: My life would have never evolved to where it is now without your support, and I am so lucky to have you in my life. I love you so much.

My yoga path began years ago because of the encouragement of Tim Aitken, a wonderful healer, who said one day I would write a book. I put that out of my head, but had many people along my path encourage me to do just that.

My first yoga teachers, Alan Finger, Janice Ventresca, Drew and Joanne Kane: knowing you is what sparked the fire that continues to burn inside of me for knowledge of this incredible practice. Emily Barton first introduced me to this practice of restorative yoga. Judith Hanson Lasater filled me with the knowledge that has helped me to become the teacher that I am today, and has given me permission to cultivate the wisdom that I have gleaned from this practice and share it with others. Cora Wen, you came into my life when I was ready to have you there. You have taught me so much, and I know you will teach me more. Your friendship has been a gift. Jean Aronoff, who really increased my knowledge base of Iyengar yoga: your sharing of what you know is so selfless, and you are a true definition of teacher and friend. Gabriel Halpern and Kofi Busia: your thirst for knowledge and the passion you bring to sharing it has fed me so much, and I am forever grateful to you. And finally, I thank Marsha Wenig, with whom I studied children's yoga: She helped me to learn the most about myself, and continues to be an example of how to conduct yourself as a kind-hearted human being.

Thank you to my Om Sweet Om family. Students, teachers, and staff: without you, this book would not be possible. Thank you to my private clients who have enriched my life as a teacher and aided me in creating a book that will help others learn how to help themselves. I wish I could mention you all by name; just know you are in my heart forever.

Erica Fazzari, Lenora Gim, Ashley Kaplan, Dave Ottaviano, Ellen Edelman, Alayna Richter, Steven Grossman, and Liz Lazar, I could not have done this without you! Thank you for giving your time to be models in this book!

Dvora Troshane helped grace this book with her beautiful chakra drawings. They were the perfect addition to the book! Thank you so much for your emotional support and your incredible talent!

Thanks to my sister Leslie Kahan, who has always supported me with love, and all the friends and family who have supported me along the journey; there are too many names to mention, and I fear that I would leave someone out inadvertently. If you are my friend, you know who you are.

Thank you, my children, who have always understood that I had an underlying thirst for knowledge and a deep desire to share what I have learned with others. Alix and Daniel, you fill me with so much love.

Lastly, thank you, David Nussbaum, for encouraging me to write this book. Thank you to the entire team at Adams Media that helped bring this book to fruition, and Brianne, without whose help this book would not have happened.

INDEX

ABOUT THE AUTHOR

Gail Boorstein Grossman, E-RYT 500, CYKT, is the founder and director of Om Sweet Om Yoga in Port Washington, NY. Gail has been teaching yoga since 2000, initially to children and then adults.

Gail has practiced meditation from the age of ten years old. Little did she know that the connection she felt through meditation would spark her later interest in the physical practice of yoga. Once she fell in love with yoga, all she has ever wanted to do was share it with others.

Gail has done her children's certifications with YogaKids, Yoga for the Special Child, and Radiant Child Yoga. She has done her adult certifications with BeYoga with Alan Finger and Janice Ventresca, and Yoga Bloom with Cora Wen. Her additional training has come from Judith Hanson Lasater, Leslie Kaminoff, Gabriel Halpern, Kofi Busia, and Leslie Howard. Gail has been a part of the Port Washington yoga community since 2000. She is a member of Yoga Alliance and the International Association of Yoga Therapists.

Gail is the proud mother of two wonderful children, Alix and Daniel, who inspired her to quit the rat race in a field that no longer fed her soul and to find a career that was about creating a life. Though running a business can be difficult at times, her family and her yoga practice help her keep it together. Her greatest hope is that she can touch as many people as possible through yoga, and help them to find balance in their lives through the physical and philosophical practices that yoga provides.

CHECK OUT MORE ONLINE!

Visit us online for exclusive access to an additional stress-relieving sequence. This short series of restorative poses can be completed in fifteen minutes—whether you're at home or in the office—and provides an easy way to relax and renew.

Go to *www.adamsmedia.com/yoga_journal* **to try it out.**
Stress relief is just fifteen minutes away!

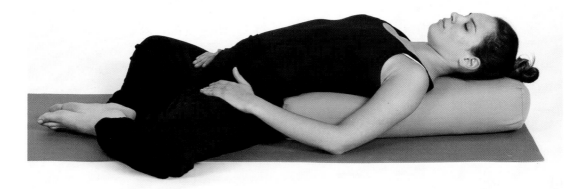